Secrets of Style

Every woman needs a business look, whether she goes to the office or has personal business.

Remember that a business look does not necessarily mean a suit.

Every woman needs
a dressed-up look.

A simple dress
can become dressy
when the
Well-Dressed Woman
knows how
to accessorize.

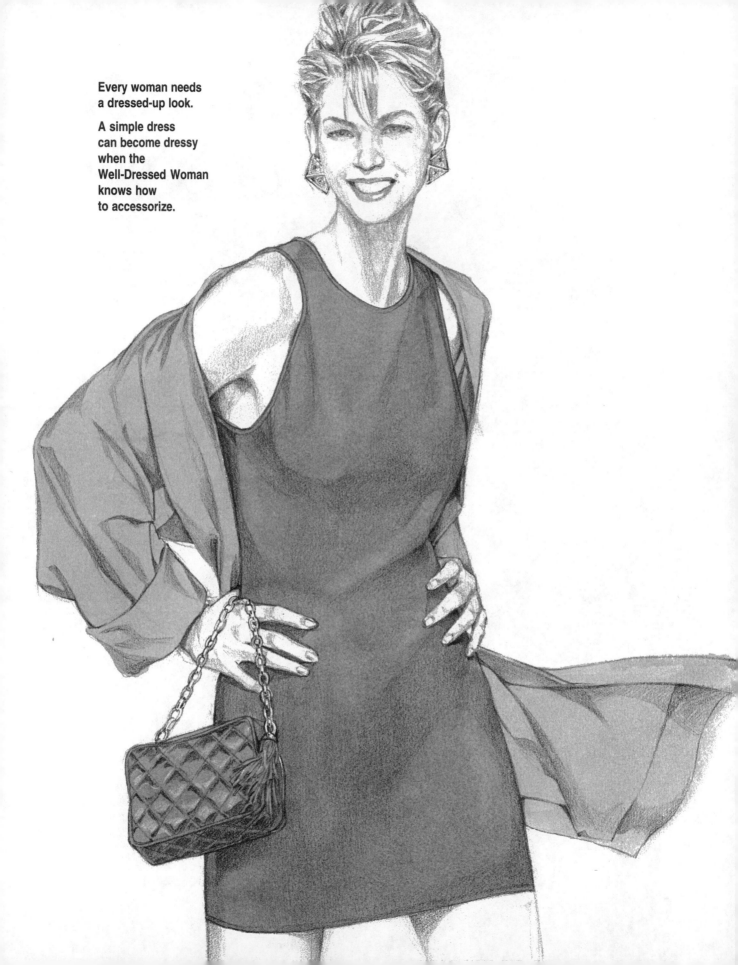

Secrets of Style

Your Personal Profile

STYLE ● BODYLINE ● WARDROBE ● COLOR ● HAIR ● MAKE-UP

Doris Pooser

Crisp Publications, Inc.

Dedicated to my Mother

Frances Wronski

for teaching me the meaning of style
and the importance of
commitment, dedication, and perseverance.

Crisp Publications, Inc.
1200 Hamilton Court
Menlo Park, CA 94025

Secrets of Style was designed by Robert Hickey. Black and white illustrations by Derek Bryant. Color Illustrations by Sachiko Kanai.

Library of Congress Cataloging in Publication Data

Doris Pooser,
Secrets of Style

ISBN 1-56052-152-X

ISBN 1-56052-152-X

ACKNOWLEDGMENTS

Secrets of Style would not have been possible without the dedication, support and commitment of many people throughout the past ten years. To all of those who have taken my courses, read my books and worked with me to demonstrate and develop the concepts presented, I thank you.

A special thanks to a few who went above and beyond in their work and support.

Marie Bowling for her efficiency, coordination and endless typing and re-typing.

Derek Bryant for so beautifully illustrating my message in his drawings and illustrations.

Phyllis Avedon for once again editing my work despite unrealistic deadlines.

Robert Hickey for his layout, design and organizational skills, but for much more -- his friendship and continued support of my color and style concepts and my mission.

My sister, Joan Molvik, for her generosity and personal support during some very difficult times.

To my son, Todd Pooser, for his expression of support in his own unique way.

To my son, Jeff Pooser, for his sensitivity, love and for always being there when I needed him.

To Wendell Minnick, for his patience, love, encouragement and belief in me and the future.

CONTENTS

Every woman
needs a casual look.

Whether it's her
everyday look
or weekend look,
it should be
current and fun.

PREFACE

Over the past ten years, thousands of men and women have been helped by using the information on color, body line and wardrobing in my *Always In Style* and *Successful Style* books and in the Secrets of Style video and workbook, and by attending seminars and consultations given by image consultants trained in the Always In Style system in more than 17 countries around the world. And yet I still get phone calls and letters asking me for more *personal* help. "Please help me *look* better *and feel* better about myself."

The requests come from all age groups, and from people at all economic and social levels: from the spunky 84-year-old who said, "Hurry, I may not have much time left," to the 13-year-old mother on welfare who had no one to ask for help.

Here are some requests for help from my files. Many of you will be able to identify with these people and their needs.

> "My children are all gone and I'm going back to work for the first time in 20 years. I'm confused by the choices of colors, styles and shapes in the stores. Where do I begin?"

> "My husband left me after 30 years of marriage for a younger woman. I have hit bottom and I need to feel better about myself."

> "I've just lost 75 pounds and I don't know where to begin with the new me."

> "I weigh 300 pounds and still want to look my best. Please help me look beautiful."

> "I've just had cancer surgery, am on chemotherapy and I need a boost."

> "I've just been promoted to a senior management position and I don't feel that I look the part. I'm so busy with my job I can't keep up with what's new, right and appropriate."

> "I'm graduating from college next month and have a limited budget. I need a professional look but want to feel like me."

"My 50th wedding anniversary is coming up next month and I want my husband to be just as proud of me as he was 50 years ago."

"I'm a single working mother with three children under 10 and take courses three nights a week toward my degree. I have little time, little money and need to look professional, but must be practical."

"I haven't felt good about myself in years — my hair is mousy, my skin is dull, I have circles under my eyes and I have big hips. Can you please help me look in the mirror and smile again?"

"I'm attractive, have a good job, love clothes and enjoy shopping. For some reason, I still have a closet full of mistakes. I just can't seem to figure out a simple solution to the problem of looking well-dressed season after season. Just as I get a few good looks together, I'm outdated again. I know there must be a logical answer. Please help."

Every one of these women wanted some simple answers, not a lot of theory or some complicated system. "Just tell me what's right for me - - and **why** — so I can continue to make the right choices. Give me a simple list of suggestions and shopping tips that will work for me, my lifestyle, my budget and my personality. And better yet, tell me where I can find these things, for real, this season!"

My mission has always been to help as many people as possible understand their own personal style and feel better about themselves. Although I have been able to accomplish this for thousands through my books and seminars, I was never completely satisfied. I wanted to really help on a more personal level.

Redefining the personal approach
About a year ago, my partner, Wendell Minnick, asked me if I'd like to write a separate book for each individual, one that would give personal advice based on their specific physical characteristics, personal preferences, needs and lifestyle.

"Of course," I replied. "All I'd have to do would be to spend a day or two with each one. A delightful dream, Wendell, but it's impossible. There's no way I could live long enough!" Fortunately for me, Wendell has this incredible belief that anything that is good is possible. "Nothing's impossible," he insisted. "You can do it and I'll help."

He asked me how much information I needed from an individual to be able to help her look better. And he asked me how I would take her step-by-step through the process of selecting the shapes, color characteristics, and design that would dramatically improve both her appearance and her confidence. I made and remade my lists and over the next year we worked together to develop the Always In Style Personal Profile database system. Thousands of women have already received their own "personalized books" — their "Personalized Profiles."

In *Secrets of Style*, I'm going to take you step-by-step through the process of developing your personal style. At the end you will have your own "Personal" book, one that will give you the information you need to look and feel wonderful.

And as each new season arrives, you will be able to update your look with the "personalized" *Always In Style Portfolio*, which not only shows you everything that will be available in the stores a full season ahead, but shows what is right for *you*.

We'll write it together, but it's really *your* book. Now, let's get started on **Secrets of Style, Your Personal Profile.** Let's discover the best possible definition of you as a woman of the 90's.

Doris Pooser

Doris Pooser
Always In Style

Author, *Secrets Of Style*

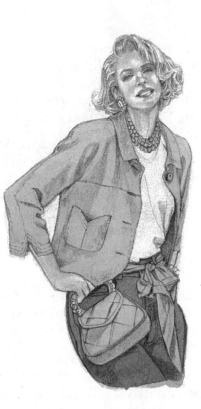

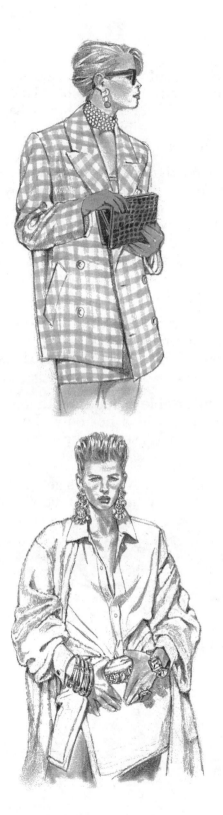

**The woman of the 90's
is an** *individual.*

**She expresses
the different facets
of her personality
at different times
because
it is honest
and fun.**

INTRODUCTION

The Image Of The Woman Of The 90's

Wherever she goes, whatever she does, she projects style and class. She seems confident, self-assured and in control. The image of the Woman of the Nineties is the image of Success.

Henry Rogers, one of America's foremost public relations experts, (with clients like Paul Newman, Sylvester Stallone, Dudley Moore, the Ford Motor Company, and Texas Instruments), says in his book, *Rogers' Rules for Success*, that "our image is our most important sales tool," and that, each and every day, every one of us is "selling ourselves." We are our own "PR Agents."

Rogers also underscores the importance of defining the word "image," which he calls "the subconscious and conscious impression we have about ourselves (our self-image) and that others have about us (our public image)."

For those who have a problem with the word image and the superficial connotations that it sometimes conjures up in today's society, he suggests replacing "image" with the phrase "True Self." We can then say that our True Self is a reflection of our self-image and public image.

Going public — looking good

Let's start by focusing on our public image, for several reasons. First, our public image can have a positive effect on our self-image. Dr. Joyce Brothers says that when we look good, we feel good about ourselves. Others respond better to us. We, in turn, begin to feel better about ourselves, which makes others respond even better to us. We create what she calls an upwardly spiraling effect that leads to both our self- and public images becoming more positive.

Second, it is easier to change our public image. It has been shown that we form a first impression within the first 30 seconds of meeting someone.

Studies at UCLA have found that 55 percent of first impressions are visual, 38 percent are based on how we speak and present ourselves, and only 7 percent on what we say.

I have found that it is far easier to change the visual, especially what we wear, than it is to change our inner feelings about ourselves.

We all have conflicts, problems and past baggage that can interfere with our inner feelings of self-confidence and control. While it is important to acknowledge our problems and take steps to overcome them, it is often a long process even to evaluate where to start.

The Woman of the 90's needs more immediate results. I know from experience — and can promise — that these immediate results help us not only to look good, but to begin to feel better about ourselves. And feeling better about ourselves definitely helps us through some of the difficult times. As I said, I speak from experience.

The woman inside: do you really know who she is?

Four years ago I was at a Career Options Conference in Anaheim, California, preparing for a presentation on the Importance of Image. Dr. Joyce Brothers was also speaking at that conference on the subject of her new book, *Successful Women*. She talked about the impossibility of being superwomen. She said that we cannot be all things — perfect wife, lover, mother, athlete, career woman — and be successful at all of these. She stressed the importance of setting priorities and learning to rid ourselves of the guilt associated with the fact that we can't be all things to all people.

This was a very important message for me that day.

I had just lost my husband after a tragic year of dealing with his undiagnosed clinical depression, my 40-year-old brother-in-law was dying of lung cancer due to asbestos exposure, and my business was falling apart, since my husband had also been my business partner, and I was trying to run an international business with little, if any, business experience. I was writing a new book, training image consultants, traveling 100,000 miles each year servicing my international contracts and trying to be the perfect mother to one son in college and one at home who was into "teenage rebellion."

At that moment I did not feel confident, self-assured or in control. I felt like a failure as a wife, mother, and businesswoman. As I listened to Dr. Brothers, I realized that I had been attempting the impossible and certainly needed to make some changes in my life. I knew that it would take time to heal the pain, to change my feelings and self-image.

I just didn't know where or how to start.

What I did know was that I needed to get up on that stage next and project style, class and confidence.

I knew that I couldn't present my True Self. I needed to present an image of success and the true self I needed to be again. I needed a crutch, a tool for survival.

And I needed it immediately.

I knew that I could project the right professional image. I was dressed in style, I could stand up tall and present the program, certainly I could speak with confidence, and I knew my subject. I, therefore, knew I would feel in control, if only during that presentation.

And one minute, one hour, one day at a time were all I could hope for at that point in my life.

I was grateful that I had developed and tested some very easy rules for assuring that my public image would be positive. I continued throughout the next several years to depend on these rules and to lean on my public image through many trying times.

Today my self-image is a little better than it was four years ago. I haven't gotten rid of all the guilt nor am I in complete control of my life, but I continue to make progress. I sometimes rely on my public image too much, when I face a difficult situation and need to boost my confidence. It's great to have a strong, effective public image to fall back on during the trying moments we all face in our lives. But it also makes it even more necessary to actively work on your self-image as you will read in Chapter Nine, Your True Self.

Reach out and touch someone

My committment is to teach as many women as possible the simple *Rules of Dressing* that have helped me and thousands of others improve our public image — and therefore our self-image — as we strive to achieve the success we all deserve.

So let's take a look at these "Simple Rules of Dressing."

Simple — but never plain

How does the Well-Dressed Woman of the 90's look? Whether she's out jogging, working at the office or enjoying a cocktail party, she always looks wonderful. People look and say things like, "she's lucky, she was born with class," or "she can afford to wear expensive clothes," or "she has beautiful features," or "lovely blond hair." They say these things because they don't understand personal style, the art of being well-dressed.

We are now going to define your personal style and help you develop the art of being well-dressed. *A woman who projects personal style is a well-dressed woman.* She projects her *personal* style in the way she looks.

What is your definition of a Well-Dressed woman? How would you describe her?

I often hear things like, "she's put-together" or "she's neat," or "she wears her right colors," or "she's coordinated."

All of these descriptions are appropriate, but they are generalities. How do we become "put-together"? Coordinated? We need some easy rules to give us the immediate steps for instant success.

My definition of a well-dressed woman provides simple guidelines for success.

The Well-Dressed Woman wears clothes, accessories, and makeup that:

1) **Complement her physically —**
   they complement her shape,
   proportion and coloring;

2) **Express her personality —**
   who she is inside as well as out;

3) **Are appropriate for the occasion —**
   we all need the right clothes,
   whether for day, work or play;

4) **Are current and fashionable —**
   wherever she goes she looks wonderful.

As we work together through the easy steps in developing your personal style, you will be writing your own personal profile. I have left blanks at the end of each section for you to use in filling in your personal details. At the end of the book there is a personal data summary form for you to complete.

To assure that you will be using the information in the following pages effectively, take a few minutes to review the glossary on page 118 and fill in the questionnaire on pages 119-120.

There are many correct answers to each question. It is Okay if you are unable to fill in all of the blanks.

Once you have finished reading *Secrets Of Style* and have completed your personal style profile, you can review *my* answers to the questionnaire that are given on page 102. It is always exciting to see your new point of view after learning a few easy concepts!

GLOSSARY

1. **Fashion** - The way of dressing that is considered the best at a given time. It is a mirror image of what is happening in the world today. The most updated and current clothes and accessories seen first on the runways, then in magazines and *Women's Wear Daily*, and finally available in the stores and boutiques for the consumer to buy.

2. **Trend** is a specific theme or style, interpreted by most designers, which will be current and available in stores for several seasons.

3. **A fad** is a specific theme or style which few designers interpret and which usually dies before the end of its first season.

4. **Style** is the unique manner in which every individual understands, interprets and applies all of the available *fashion* to herself. *Each person must learn to develop her own style by understanding the relationship of clothing to her own physical coloring and shape. Your personal style is the total reflection of who you are.*

5. **Fashion Portfolio** is a complete, up-to-date fashion resource available twice a year. It is fully illustrated; contains current fashions, colors, fabrics, themes, silhouettes and wardrobe plans for each body type.

6. **Line** - an infinite number of points with a direction. A line can be straight or curved or some combination.

7. **Body lines** - face and body shapes can be described by geometric shapes and can be placed on a graph from the straightest to the most curved. (Body line categories: Straight, Soft Straight, Straight Soft, and Curved). Body lines are determined by bone structure and the way the flesh is arranged around the bone structure.
    Soft Straight was previously referred to as *Soft-Straight I.*
    Straight Soft was previously referred to as *Soft-Straight II.*

8. **Silhouette line** - the exterior line of a garment.

9. **Detail lines** - pockets, trim, epaulets, shoulder seams, etc.

10. **Clothing lines** - include both silhouette and detail lines.

11. **Scale** - the relationship of the size of a garment or accessory to the individual's size.

12. **High-fashion look** - an exaggeration of line, scale and/or detail. The latest look, often a style, that is just coming in on the fashion cycle.

QUESTIONNAIRE

Each of these questions has many correct answers. Some of our answers are on page 102.

1. List the four ways in which your clothes can complement you physically.

a) _____

b) _____

c) _____

d) _____

2. How can you express your personality in the way you dress?

a) _____

b) _____

c) _____

d) _____

3. List the different occasions and types of clothes you need for your lifestyle.

Occasion	Types of Clothes

4. List three ways to help you determine your wardrobe needs.

a) _____

b) _____

c) _____

5. List a basic capsule wardrobe of 10 to 14 pieces that will serve all of your needs. _____

_____

_____

6. How can you quickly change a casual outfit to make it appropriate for work or give it a dressy look? _____

_____

_____

7. List four ways in which you can update your look each season.

a) _____

b) _____

c) _____

d) _____

8. Do you like wearing black, or want to but haven't felt confident in black? How can you wear black or any other fashion color in a way that is complementary to you? _____

_____

_____

9. List four makeup tips that can change your look from day to evening.

a) _____

b) _____

c) _____

d) _____

10. Describe your personal style. _____

_____

_____

_____

It's Okay
if you cannot
answer all these questions
at this time.

Consider the ideas presented
and look forward
to learning more
about each concept
in the following
chapters.

Some of the answers
I would suggest
appear on page 102.

— Doris Pooser

Every garment
is designed
for a particular
body line.

If it doesn't fit,
it may NOT be the size,
but the shape.

Discover
your body line
so you can
choose
what's best
for you.

CHAPTER ONE

Body Line

The Well-Dressed Woman
wears clothes that complement her physically

Clothes that complement us physically enhance three aspects of ourselves —
our *shape*, *proportion* and *coloring*. They look like a natural extension of
ourselves, like they were made for us. Wouldn't it be wonderful to know that
you could always look like you had a personal dressmaker and that you
could achieve this in less time and with less money than ever before? Let's
look at each of these elements one at a time, starting with shape.

SHAPE

When we hear the word shape most women cringe a bit and start making
excuses, general or specific. "Don't talk about shapes." Or "my body is
awful." "I need to lose weight, my hips are big." "My legs are ugly." "My
nose is crooked." Rarely do we stand up straight and comfortably approach
the subject. Instead we pursue it with slight embarrassment and consider-
able caution.

This preoccupation with the "latest" perfect body results from years of
being told that some body shapes are definitely more "in style" than others
— the well-endowed "Marilyn Monroe" look of the fifties, the "Twiggy"
look of the 60's, the rounded "Madonna" look of the 80's. These stereotypes
feed our insecurities and lead us to be overly critical of our bodies.

It is important to remember that each of us was born with a unique shape:
no one is better than another. Fortunately, the woman of the 90's recognizes
the need to express her individuality. We all understand the need to be
personally fit for health reasons and are beginning to accept the fact that no
one shape is ideal.

Identifying your body line is the first step in recognizing and accepting
yourself and in learning how to select clothes that reflect your unique
qualities. We no longer need to approach the subject of our body shape with
trepidation.

Face shape

To determine your overall body line, let's start with your face shape. We are all familiar with classic shapes: heart, pear, round, oval, square, rectangle or diamond.

Saying no to the ideal oval

For years we have been told that the ideal face shape is oval and that we should select hairstyles that make our faces look less angular or less curved. I disagree! If you have a wonderful square jawline and chiseled features, play them up — that's you.

If you have a curved face with big round eyes, why try to make your face look like just another "almost" oval face? Instead of trying to make our face shape look "almost" oval and always missing the mark, it is better to identify our individual face shape and work with it — to enhance the angles or to complement the soft contours. Once you identify your face shape, you will be able to select necklines, lapels and jewelry that are flattering to you.

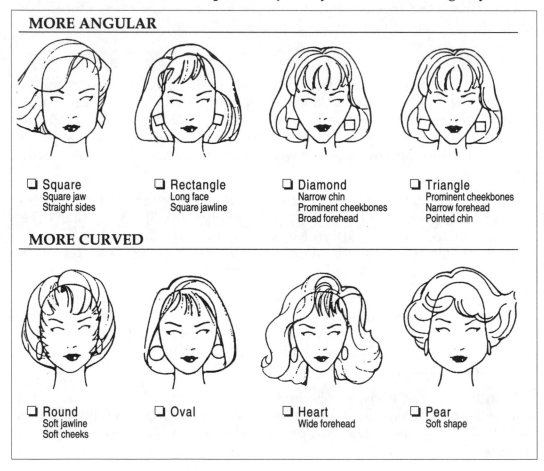

MORE ANGULAR

❏ **Square**
Square jaw
Straight sides

❏ **Rectangle**
Long face
Square jawline

❏ **Diamond**
Narrow chin
Prominent cheekbones
Broad forehead

❏ **Triangle**
Prominent cheekbones
Narrow forehead
Pointed chin

MORE CURVED

❏ **Round**
Soft jawline
Soft cheeks

❏ **Oval**

❏ **Heart**
Wide forehead

❏ **Pear**
Soft shape

Since many of us have face shapes that are a combination of angles and curves, look carefully at your overall face shape and decide whether you see more softness or more angles.

Remember, we are not looking for an exact label (square or round), but more for the overall shape. Look at the exterior shape as well as your features to identify a soft contoured shape or one with more defined angles.

Look in the mirror. Stand back. Do not try to figure out a specific shape, but look for an overall impression. Look especially at your jawline.

Consider: do you see more angles or more curves? Look for one or more of the following:

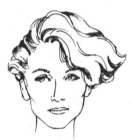
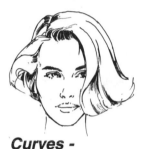

Angles	*Curves -*
Square jawline	Softness in overall look
Pointed chin	Contoured shape
Prominent cheekbones	Round cheeks
Straightness of sides	Curved jawline
Angular features	Soft chin
Straight forehead	Round eyes
Tapered or slender nose	Arched eyebrows
	Full lips

Now select your face shape.

My face shape is: ❑ ANGULAR
❑ CONTOURED

Note: The shapes of your earrings should enhance your face shape. Do not repeat your face shape. However, choose somewhat angular shapes if your face is angular and a soft shape if your face is more curved. You probably have favorite earrings. They are likely to be the ones that look the best on you because they create a balance and harmony with your face shape. I am not suggesting that you emphasize extremes unless you want a dramatic look like the punk style of the 80's. Just enhance your face shape.

Body Shape

Look at the four body lines on page 29 and their corresponding body line symbols. These symbols will be used throughout the book and are used in the *Always In Style Portfolio* Fashion Forecast to help identify garments that have the same or similar shape as your body line. Take time to think about the celebrities listed and their shapes. Would you put the same dress on Nancy Reagan and Elizabeth Taylor? Martina Navratilova and Jane Pauley? Of course not. Nancy Reagan looks better in straighter silhouettes, Elizabeth Taylor in more curved or shaped garments. Where do you fit along this line? Are you more straight or more curved, or are you a combination?

Now let's identify your body shape. Is it more rounded or more straight? Remember, weight has nothing to do with your body line. It is your bone structure and the way the flesh is arranged around your bones that determine your body line. Look for a softer shape or a more linear form. Once you understand your bodyline, your clothes will fit you better and look like a natural extension of you.

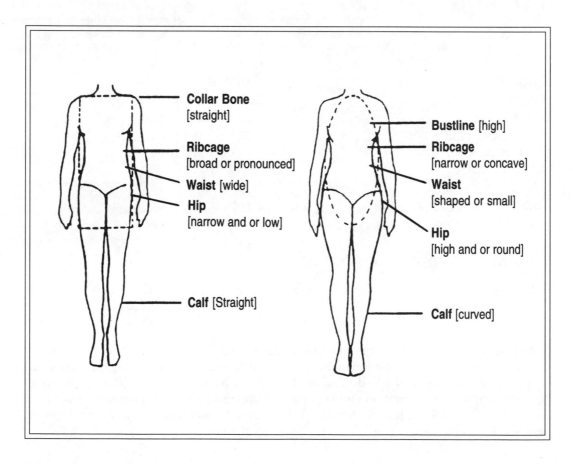

Collar Bone [straight]

Ribcage [broad or pronounced]

Waist [wide]

Hip [narrow and or low]

Calf [Straight]

Bustline [high]

Ribcage [narrow or concave]

Waist [shaped or small]

Hip [high and or round]

Calf [curved]

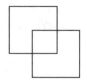

STRAIGHT

A straight body shape will project *some* of the following:
- ✓ Straight shoulders
- ✓ Prominent collarbones
- ✓ Wide midriff - thick waist
- ✓ Long torso
- ✓ Narrow hip - (may have protruding buttocks)
- ✓ Flat hips and/or stomach
- ✓ Straight legs
- ✓ Straight stance
- ✓ Straight walk
- ✓ Low bustline
- ✓ Low hipbones
- ✓ Waist, midriff, hip similar in size

Remember, a straight body line is still feminine. You have a waist, bust and hipline. Your waist may not be small and your hipline is probably not rounded, although it may be broad. Look for an overall shape so that you will be able to select clothing that looks like it was made for you — like it fits your shape. A round, curved seam will not fit correctly on a straight hipline.

CURVED

A curved body shape will project *some* of the following:
- ✓ Soft shoulder line
- ✓ Round bust *(often full but not necessarily)*
- ✓ Small or tapered rib cage
- ✓ High hipbones
- ✓ Small waist (relative to hip size)
- ✓ Round hip
- ✓ Tilted hip stance
- ✓ High bustline
- ✓ Roundness of flesh
- ✓ Round stomach
- ✓ Curved legs
- ✓ Hip movement when walking

Remember, a curved body is not necessarily an overweight body. It projects a roundness — a tailored, straight seam does not fit a curved hip properly. It pulls and gaps.

Now select your body shape.

My body shape is: ❑ STRAIGHT   ❑ CURVED

Your **Body Line** is defined as a combination of your
face shape and your **body shape.**

It is now possible to identify your body line category by using your face shape and body shape combination. Notice the body line symbols indicate where you are curved and where you are straight.

STRAIGHT BODY LINE
angular face, straight body

STRAIGHT-SOFT BODY LINE
angular face, curved body

SOFT-STRAIGHT BODY LINE
contoured face, straight body

CURVED BODY LINE
contoured face, curved body

My Body Line category is:
- ❏ **STRAIGHT**
- ❏ **STRAIGHT SOFT**
- ❏ **SOFT STRAIGHT**
- ❏ **CURVED**

NOTE: Some of you may be having difficulty determining whether your face is more contoured or more angular, you may see a combination of angles and curves. In this case, you will be better in one of the **SOFT-STRAIGHT** categories. To decide which of the SOFT & STRAIGHT combinations best describes you, look at your body shape again.

To determine SOFT STRAIGHT or STRAIGHT SOFT:

1. If your body is more curved, play up the angles in your face —
   choose **STRAIGHT SOFT** as your body line.

2. If your body is more straight, play up the softness in your face —
   choose **SOFT STRAIGHT** as your body line.

My body line is:
- ❏ **SOFT STRAIGHT**
- ❏ **STRAIGHT SOFT**

Remember that you are an individual. Use your body line category and suggested shapes as guidelines only. You may be able to use some shapes from a second group that is more like your primary body line category.

Try to place your body line somewhere on the graph between straight and curved. For confirmation of your body line, look at the silhouette shapes for each body line type in Chapter Two. See which shapes tend to fit you best or which you are most comfortable wearing. We are usually most comfortable with what is right for us.

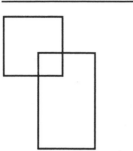 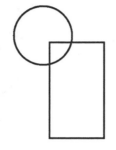 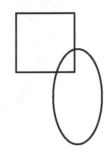 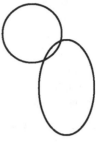

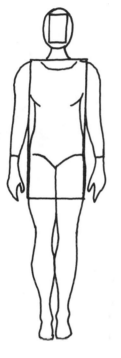 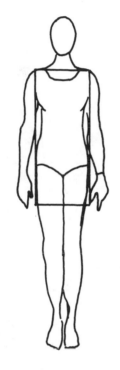 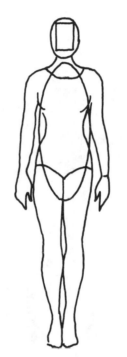 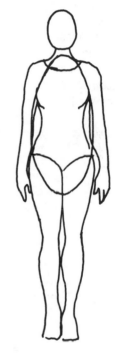

Straight
Angular face
Straight body

Straight Examples
Jackie Onassis
Nancy Reagan
Nancy Kissinger
Martina Navratilova

Soft Straight
Contoured face
Straight body

Soft-Straight Examples
Yoko Ono
The Queen Mother
Katie Couric

Straight Soft
Angular face
Curved body

Straight-Soft Examples
Linda Evans
Raquel Welch
Barbara Walters
Catherine Crier

Curved
Contoured face
Curved body

Curved Examples
"Fergie"
Elizabeth Taylor
Jane Pauley
Hillary Clinton

If you gain
or lose 25
or even 50 pounds,
your basic body line
will not change.

If your body line
is straight,
it will remain straight.

If your body line
is curved,
it will remain curved.

Selecting clothing
with the same
or similar shape
as your body line
is the first step
in becoming a
well-dressed
woman.

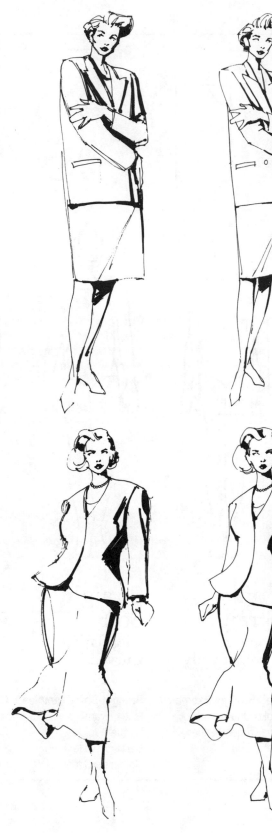

CHAPTER TWO

Clothing & Accessories

For clothes to look like a natural extension of you and to complement you, your clothing lines must follow (be the same as or similar to) your body line. Review the silhouette shapes and notice how the neckline area should complement your face shape and how the body of the garment should look — like it fits your body shape.

It really is very logical when you consider how my body line concept relates to the old cliche "You can't put a square peg in a round hole."

So many women have called me to say how much better they look, how much thinner, and how pleased they are with this new yet really old concept. Many have pointed out that for years they were told to do the opposite — to wear a soft gathered floral dress if they had a straight shape to look more curved, or a boxy tailored style to "cover" the curves. Most have never been comfortable trying to change or cover their shapes but didn't know why.

Finding the best in "you"

I once had a client who was six feet tall and large-boned with a very straight body line. She drove racing cars for a living but had many social functions to attend. Because she was in a male-dominated profession and not petite, she thought she would look more feminine by dressing in floral chiffon dresses for her banquets.

She arrived for a consultation with an armful of expensive, pretty dresses, knowing something was wrong. I showed her how a simple silk crepe or satin shift dress or tunic over silk pants made her look more feminine, and in fact thinner, by keeping her silhouette straight and using a dressy fabric. She had found the secret of enhancing her own body shape and then and there began developing her personal style.

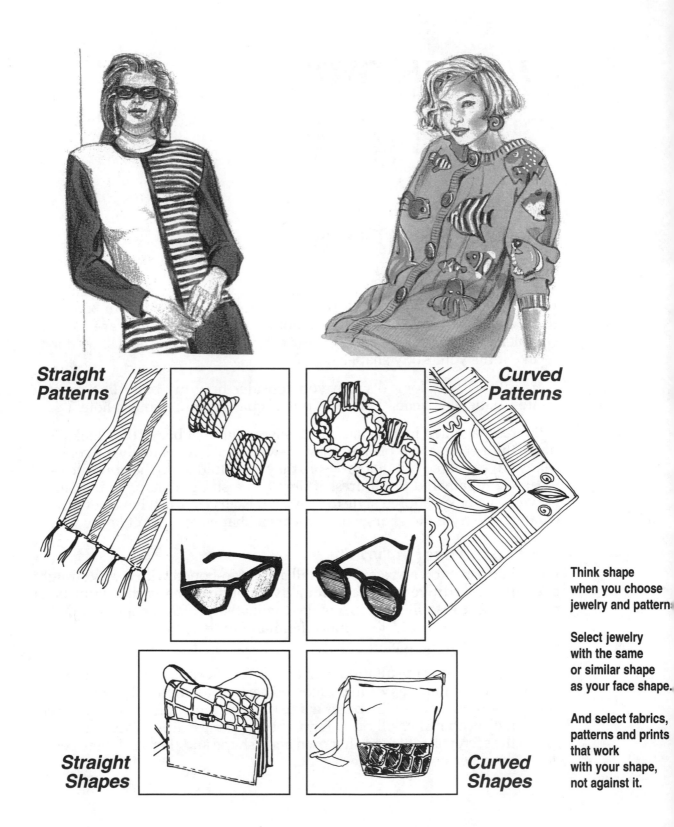

**Straight
Patterns**

**Curved
Patterns**

Think shape
when you choose
jewelry and pattern.

Select jewelry
with the same
or similar shape
as your face shape.

And select fabrics,
patterns and prints
that work
with your shape,
not against it.

**Straight
Shapes**

**Curved
Shapes**

Think shape when you choose jewelry and patterns

Select jewelry with the same or similar shape as your face shape. And select fabrics, patterns and prints that work *with* this shape, not against it. When selecting patterns and prints, you will notice that geometric patterns and prints are better with straighter styles. Paisleys, swirls and florals are better with more rounded or curved shapes.

Shapes everyone can wear

There are a few shapes and designs that can be worn by everyone since the line is a softened line — neither too straight nor too curved. Adding the correct shape jewelry, accessories and patterns in the shape that's correct for your will give you the desired overall effect either more straight or more curved.

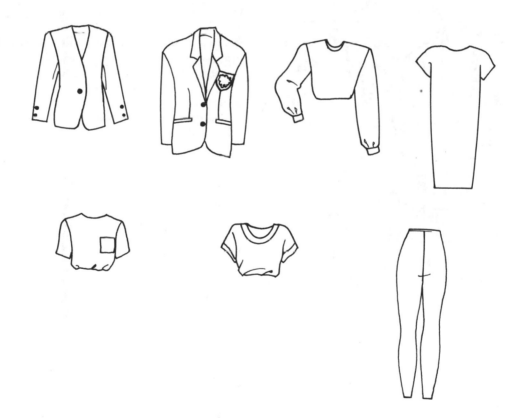

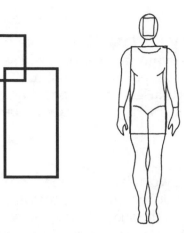

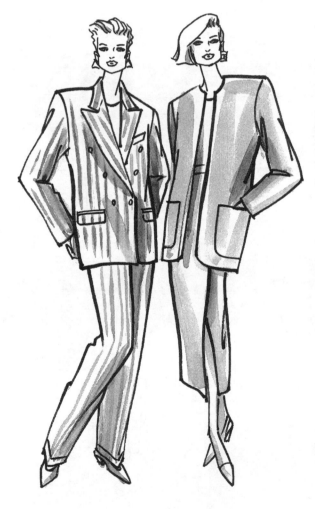

Straight
Angular face
Straight body

Straight Silhouette Lines
☐ Crisp, straight closings
☐ Angular and asymmetrical detail
☐ Well-defined shoulders
☐ Straight jacket and skirt hemlines
☐ Little or no waist emphasis
☐ Tailored lines

Straight Details
It is important for the details used on clothing to be consistent with the silhouette lines:

Darts: Long straight, sharply defined or no darts.

Seams: Well-defined seam lines, topstitching, contrasting piping, braid or trim.

Pleats: Pressed-down, stitched-down, asymmetrical, unpressed pleats.

Sleeves: Set-in, straight pleats at shoulder, square shoulder pads, tapered sleeves, crisp puffs.

Lapels: Notched, pointed, peaked or no lapels, edge-to-edge.

Pockets: Well-defined, square, piped, slashed.

Necklines: Square, boat, jewel, contrasting trim, V, mandarin, turtleneck.

Fabrics: Tightly woven fabrics, little or no texture

Accessories: Jewelry, bags, scarves, buckles, belts, handbags and shoes: Choose angular shapes scaled to your body size and bone structure.

Eyeglass Frames: Choose frames with some straightness across the top or with squared edges to complement the angles in your face.

These silhouettes complement a Straight body line.

Notice the straight exterior lines and crisp, clean details. Choose geometric patterns, and linear details.

Although all of the silhouettes reflect a straightness, some will be more complementary than others, depending on individual proportions.

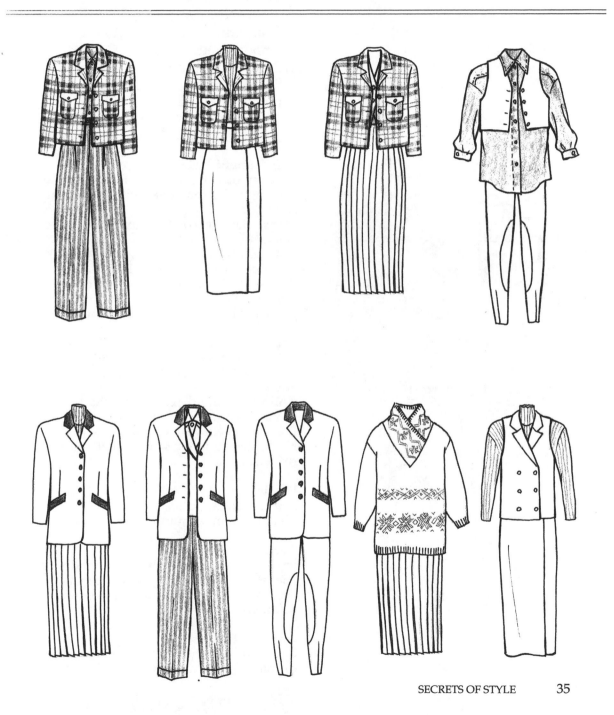

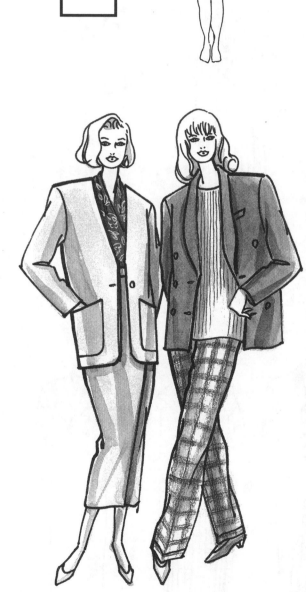

Soft Straight
Contoured face, Straight body

Soft-Straight Silhouette Lines
❑ Combination of straight and smooth lines
❑ Soft lines around face
❑ Straighter silhouettes below bustline
❑ Unconstructed shapes that are neither all straight nor all curved

Soft-Straight Details
It is important for the details used on clothing to be consistent with the silhouette lines:
Darts: Use in combination with eased detail.
Seams: Straight with unconstructed look; self-topstitching works well.
Pleats: Pressed down with soft fabric, unpressed.
Sleeves: Set-in, raglan, dolman, rounded shoulder pads.
Lapels: Notched with round edges, notched soft fabric, shawl, bias, no lapel with curved closing, rounded, dropped notch.
Collars: Rolled, cowl, notched with rounded corners.
Pockets: Patch with round bottoms, flap.
Necklines: Curved, scoop, cowl, draped, ruffled, jewel.

Fabrics
Soft woven fabric
Medium to maximum texture

Accessories
Jewelry, scarves, belts, buckles, handbags and shoes: Choose softened geometric shapes, unconstructed or constructed of soft material.

Eyeglass Frames
Choose frames with round or curved edges to complement the curves in your face.

Straight Soft

These silhouettes complement a Soft-Straight body line.

Notice the soft detailing in collars, necklines, and shoulder treatments. This softness is often carried through to the bust line. Straighter lines appear in the torso, waist, and hip area.

The combination of the softened top and straight body create a unique silhouette.

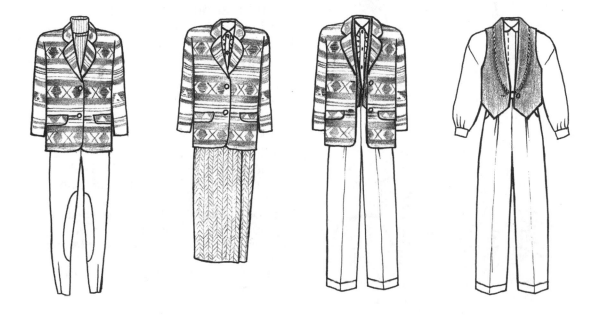

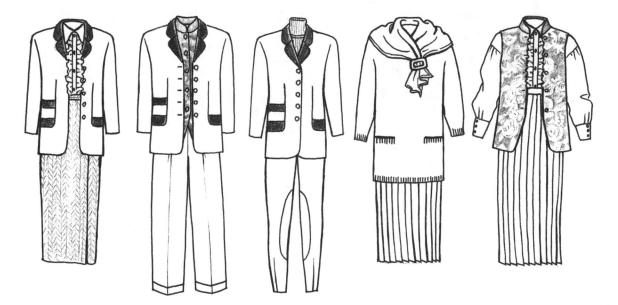

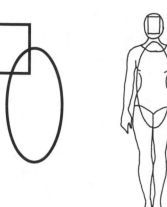

Angular face, Curved body

Straight-Soft Silhouette Lines

- ❑ Combinations of straight and smooth lines
- ❑ Crisp, straight lines around face and shoulders
- ❑ Waist emphasis
- ❑ Unconstructed and wrap shapes that are neither all straight nor all curved

Straight-Soft Details
It is important for the details used on clothing to be consistent with the silhouette lines:

Darts: Soft gathers, soft pleats, eased, used in combination with straight details.

Seams: Straight with shaping at or below waist.

Pleats: Soft, unpressed, gathered, eased.

Sleeves: Set-in, squared-off pads or pleated detail.

Collars: Notched, pointed, stand-up, straight.

Lapels: Notched or peaked with soft fabric, no lapels.

Pockets: Slashed, flap, square with soft fabric.

Necklines: Boat, jewel, V, mandarin, turtleneck.

Fabrics:
Soft woven fabrics
Medium to maximum texture

Accessories
Jewelry, scarves, buckles, belts, handbags and shoes: Choose softened geometric shapes, unconstructed or constructed of soft material.

Eyeglass Frames
Choose frames with some straightness across the top or squarish to complement the angles in your face.

Curved

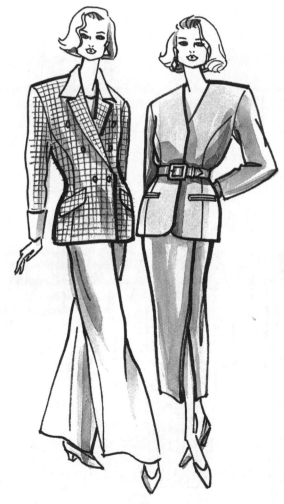

These silhouettes complement a Straight-Soft body line.

Notice the crisp, clean lines around the face and shoulder area. The body silhouette is then softened with shaped waist treatments, or soft flowing styles to create the perfect mix of two shapes.

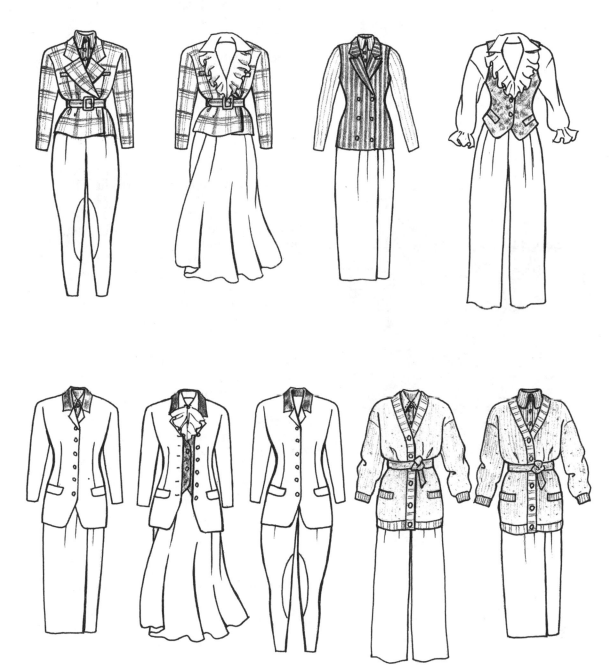

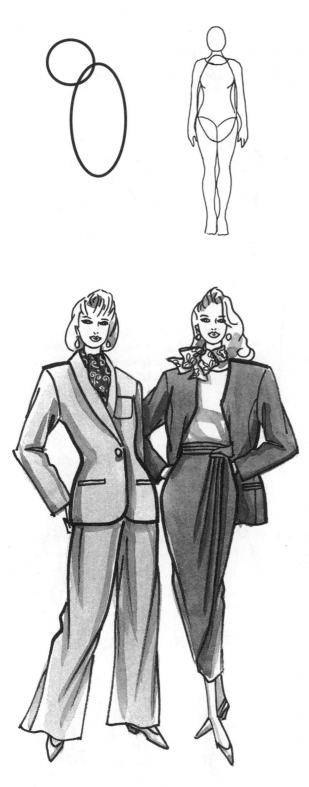

Contoured face
Curved body

Curved Silhouette Lines
- ❏ Smooth, sleek curves on closings and lapels
- ❏ Soft skirts
- ❏ Rounded hemlines
- ❏ Eased, flowing with movement to fall with the curves, not against them

Curved Details
It is important for the details used on clothing to be consistent with the silhouette lines:

Darts: Soft gathers, soft pleats, eased.
Seams: Curved seams, no topstitching, or fine topstitching, eased.
Pleats: Soft, unpressed, gathered.
Sleeves: Gathered, drop-shoulder, raglan, dolman, full and billowy.
Lapels: Rounded, curved, shawl, bias, no lapels with curved closings.
Collars: Round, rolled, cowl, notched with rounded edges or drop notch.
Pockets: Flap, rounded, set-in.
Necklines: Round, scoop, cowl, draped, ruffled, jewel, flounced.

Fabrics
Softly woven fabric and patterns
Little or no texture

Accessories
Jewelry, scarves, belts, buckles, handbags and shoes: Choose rounded, contoured and softly constructed shapes.

Eyeglass Frames
Choose frames with round or curved edges to complement the curves in your face.

Theses silhouettes complement a Curved body line.

Notice the softness in the collar and shoulder treatment. Either waist emphasis or soft flowing styles create the soft silhouette so complementary to the curved body.

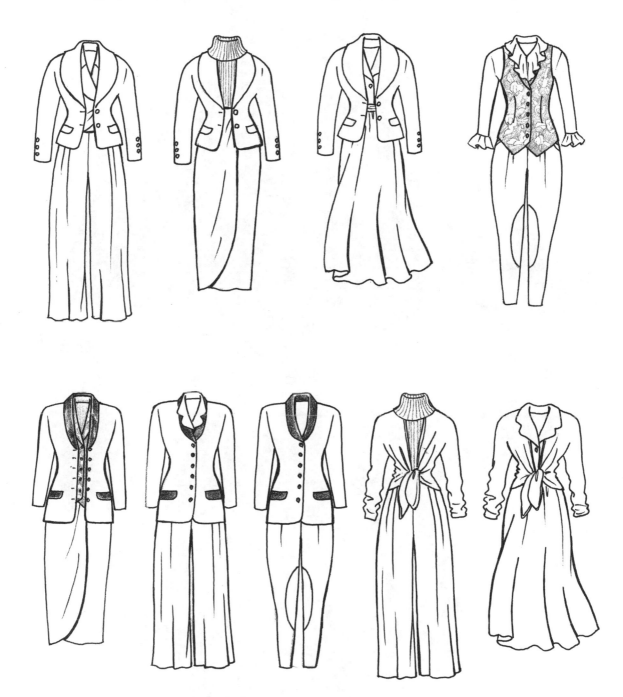

Proportion means
wearing clothes
that complement
your body line
and therefore
make
minor figure
concerns
disappear.

CHAPTER THREE

Proportion

Minor Figure Concerns

Now that we have identified your body line and have identified silhouette shapes to complement your body line, you're likely to have discovered that you have fewer figure concerns than you thought. Those of you who have a Straight or Soft Straight body line do *not* have a thick waist problem. You just have a thicker waist than someone with a more curved body line. That is your shape and body structure. Even if you devote your life to diet and exercise you cannot change your bone structure and the way your flesh is genetically programmed to frame your bones. A full ribcage is a full ribcage. A rounded tummy is a rounded tummy.

With my curved body at my thinnest, I still have a protruding stomach. More so when I do not stick to my exercise but when I do, it's still not flat. When you select clothing with less waist emphasis, a thick waist stops being an issue. When you select clothes with waist emphasis and curved hip shape, a fuller stomach appears to protrude less.

Downplaying your negatives

Those of you who have rounded or full hips do not necessarily have a hip problem. When you select shapes that are more curved or rounded, you find that your clothes fit better and de-emphasize the curve. It is only when we try to put that "square peg in a round hole" that we have a real problem.

We often hear bodies referred to as pear-shaped. Pear refers to a curved body shape that is heavier at the bottom and narrow at the top. By following suggestions for narrow or sloping shoulders and big hips, you can build or extend the shoulder line with shoulder pads or details and downplay the hip.

There are, however, individuals with straight body lines who also have wide hips and narrow shoulders. This shape is often referred to as a triangle. The hip is wide but not necessarily round; the overall shape is less curved. The same techniques — building the shoulder and de-emphasizing the hips — apply. Use a softer, more rounded shoulder pad for a curved face, and a straighter or more square pad or epaulet for an angular face.

Work with your body line, then make corrections for any minor figure concerns to create balance, harmony and eye-pleasing proportion.

The few minor figure concerns that may need some extra treatment can be managed by making some small adjustments to create balance and a more pleasing proportion. Use the following suggestions to make the minor adjustments you may need, beginning with a look in the mirror to recognize your uniqueness.

Remember, we need to work with our shape and do **as most men do** when they look in the mirror. Regardless of how they look, they tend to give themselves a pat on the back, hold their head up and say to themselves, "You handsome devil."

It's time we women look in the mirror, hold our heads up and say, "You beautiful woman."

Suggestions for Minor Figure Concerns

Once you have determined your body line and identified some of your best clothing shapes, you can make some easy adjustments to balance minor figure problems. Remember to maintain your correct clothing and silhouette shapes based on your body line. Use the following suggestions to make adjustments, using only those that apply to specific shapes that are complementary to your body lines.

Large Bust

Wear:	**Avoid:**
Open necklines	Horizontal detail
Long sleeves	High necklines
Dolman sleeves	Pockets at bustline
Loose-fitting garments	High waistbands
Vertical detail	Tight-fitting garments
	Large patterns on top

Small Bust

Wear:	**Avoid:**
Textures and/or tweeds	Low necklines
Horizontal lines	High waists
Layering	
Pockets at bustline	
Loose-fitting garments	
Bows or ties	

Cowls or turtlenecks
Gathers or pleats at bustline for fullness
Embroidery and details at bustline
Yokes
Prints on top

Long Neck

Wear:
Scarves tied at neckline (in a style that complements your face shape)
Necklines with bows or ties
Choker necklaces
High collars

Avoid:
Low necklines unless accompanied by scarves or jewelry

Short Neck

Wear:	**Avoid:**
V or U necklines	High neck treatments
Open collars	Large necklaces
Bows and scarves tied low	Scarves tied high at neck
Long necklaces	

Long Waist

Wear:
Empire and high-rise waists
Wide belts
Belts the same color as fabric below the waist

Short Waist

Wear:	**Also Wear:**
Yokes on skirts	Medium to narrow belts
Dropped waists	Belts the same color as tops
No waistband	

Short Legs

Wear:	**Avoid**
Short skirts	Border designs at hemlines
High-waisted skirts and slacks	Long, pleated skirts
Cropped trousers	*(allow some leg to show)*
Hose to match shoes and hemline	Cuffs on trousers

Long Legs

Wear:
Short skirts at or below knee
Long pleated skirts
Cuffs on trousers
Interest at leg area using pleats and border designs
Dropped yokes

Avoid:
Very short skirts
Cropped trousers

Broad Shoulders

Wear:
Small or no shoulder pads
Halters
Raglan sleeves
V or scoop neck with
    softened shoulder treatments

Avoid:
Epaulets
Details at shoulder
Boat necklines

Narrow Shoulders

Wear:
Shoulder pads
Cap sleeves
Boat necks
Horizontal details at shoulder
Dropped shoulder seams
Wide necklines
Gathers or pleats at shoulders

Avoid:
Raglan or dolman sleeves
V or U necklines
Halters

Large Hips

Wear:
Dresses with loose belts
Overblouses with dropped belt
Stitched-down pleats
Center seams or inverted pleats
Solid, deep colors on bottom
Prints, light or bright colors on top
Stripes

Avoid:
Pockets at hipline
Details at hipline
Jackets and tops that end
        at widest part of hip
Prints or patterned skirts and slacks
Light colors below the waist

Proper Fit

Clothes that complement us physically also fit properly

A final touch in having your clothes complement your shape is proper fit. Will your clothes look inexpensive or will they look elegant? Proper fit can make the difference. For an elegantly loose fit, review the following *Proper Fit Chart*.

BLOUSES, TOPS AND JUMPERS
* The seam of set-in sleeves should be located outside the shoulder bone.
* Cuffs on long sleeves should be on the wrist bone when the arm is bent.
* Sleeve width should allow at least 1" of double fabric when pinched away from your upper arm.
* There should be 2" of double fabric on either side of your diaphragm for styles that require blousing. Buttons should never pull opened.
* Body-conscious styles, bodysuits and fitted waists should allow for 1" of extra fabric.

JACKETS AND COATS
* Shoulder should be a minimum of 1" wider than the shoulder bone.
* When buttoned, the coat should allow for blouses, jumpers and tops and not pull across the shoulder, hip or bustline.
* Sleeve length should allow for 1/2" of blouse sleeve to show.
* There should be no pull across the back.
* Pockets must remain closed, pleats and darts must lie flat.

SKIRTS
* Pleats should never pull open.
* There should be no creasing or pulling across the break of the leg.
* Skirts should not ride up when you sit down.
* Straight skirts should not curve under at buttocks.
* Waistband should allow for two fingers to be inserted into the side.
* There should be at least 1" of double fabric when you pinch the skirt out from hip line (about 6" below waistline).
* Thighs and panty line must not show.
* Skirt should be easy to turn around body.

PANTS
* Pleats must remain closed; zipper and closing must lie flat.
* Pant legs should not curve under at the buttocks.
* Pockets should not gape.
* You should be able to pinch 1" to 1-1/2" of double fabric from hip line.
* Panty line must not show.
* Waistband should allow for two fingers to be inserted into the side.

What color
would you
choose?

We all
have
our best
colors,
but
there are
some colors
that
complement
everyone.

CHAPTER FOUR

Coloring

Now that we have determined your body line, identified the shapes that correctly complement your unique shape, and made adjustments for fit and proportion, let's take the next step and look at your coloring.

Over the years, there have been many color systems devised to determine an individual's best colors. In many cases, they have been helpful and they have certainly made us aware of color and its importance in determining our best look. However, many of these systems have been limiting, forcing us to choose all cool or all warm colors, or all light or all deep, and suggesting that we stay with these colors forever.

Taking the mystery out of color choices

After years of working with many color systems and color-draping thousands of people, I have developed a set of very simple color *guidelines* that identify some basic complementary colors based on eye color, hair color and skintone. And these guidelines offer flexibility — they take your personal preferences into consideration and enable you to update your colors each season based on current fashion colors and combinations.

These guidelines, which are now used by thousands of individuals throughout the world, have been substantiated by cosmetic and skin care labs, hair product companies and dermatologists in their scientific and laboratory studies.

Color facts to be noted:

☞We do not have to decide between all warm and all cool colors. There are many colors — like true red, true green, turquoise, violet, coral-pink, periwinkle blue, gray, navy and teal — that can be considered neither all warm nor all cool. These colors can be worn by everyone. They are universal colors.

☞Many of us have coloring that is a combination of warm and cool characteristics, which makes it possible for us to wear both cool and warm colors, depending on our mood, our preference and the season. You will often find that your skintone will reflect the color you are wearing, creating a slightly warmer or cooler tone which can be further enhanced by makeup in a complementary tone.

☛Just as it is important to identify our basic body shapes, we need to recognize our basic color characteristics. We can then wear colors in ways that complement our unique coloring by creating a balance and harmony.

Balance and harmony

Let's consider what we mean by balance and harmony. Close your eyes for a moment and picture several women walking into the room.

1.	Mary has dark hair, dark brown eyes and an olive complexion. What is she wearing? Do you see her in pastels? Probably not. She is more likely to be wearing black, white, red — deeper colors.

2.	Kathy has blond hair, blue eyes and a light complexion. What is she wearing? Dark heavy tones? She is more likely to be wearing gray, periwinkle blue, rose or coral-pink.

3.	Susan has red hair, olive green eyes and freckles. Most of us recognise colors like gold, rust, green — *earthtones* — complement her vivid hair and rich coloring.

4.	How about Judy? She has porcelain skin, dark hair and bright blue eyes. You would not picture her in dull or drab colors. How about bright blue, violet, clear pink or red?

5.	Phyllis has ash blond hair and dark brown eyes, a unique combination that projects some strength but with softness. Picture her in neutrals like taupe and beige, blended with rose or a soft teal. Bright primary tones just don't seem harmonious with her distinctive coloring.

6.	June has salt and pepper hair, soft brown eyes and beige skin. Grays, whites and blues obviously complement her coloring. Camel from head-to-toe would fight with her gray hair.

Breaking the old color rules

Without strict *seasonal* categories, definitions or rules, it becomes easier to identify complementary colors when we select those of the same (or similar) depth, brightness or undertone as our personal coloring. But can we wear other colors that project a different characteristic? Can Kathy, with her light blond hair and blue eyes, wear deep or bright colors? Of course, but she must have a dramatic personality, use more makeup and/or exaggerate her accessories to balance the strong color next to her light coloring. A conservative blond with fair skin who wears little makeup can be overpowered by black or deep colors and is better in gray or softer shades.

Let's look at your unique coloring, identify some dominant basic colors that complement your coloring and discover how you can wear all colors in a unique and flattering way. Once you've learned how, you can then identify your best shades from the new fashion colors each season.

Color Characteristics

Before we look at how specific colors relate to your personal coloring, it is important to understand the characteristics of color.

Undertone — all colors are made up of three primary colors — red, blue and yellow. Yellow is warm, blue is cool and red is neither cool nor warm, but "in-between." As we add yellow, we get a warmer tone; as we add blue we get a cooler tone. Green is a mixture of yellow (warm) and blue (cool). If we mix equal yellow and blue, the green we get is neither warm nor cool but "in-between." And there are many other colors that are or appear to the human eye to be "in-between."

Examples:
orange-red............................warm
blue-red ....cool
true red ....in-between

Depth - how dark or light a color may be. Some colors can be defined as deep, others as light and some are in-between. It becomes a judgment call as to whether blue denim is dark or light.

Examples:
burgundy .... deep
pink......................................light
rose......................................in-between

Brightness - how vivid or muted (soft) a color may be. Some colors are very bright, others very drab or dusty and some in-between.

Examples:
fuchsia .... bright
mauve..................................muted
rose ....in-between

All colors have these three characteristics.

When we look at a color we often see one characteristic first. We call this the *most dominant color characteristic*. I have defined dominant characteristics as:

Deep
Colors that are medium to deep in range and are neither too warm nor too cool. Navy, forest green, true red, charcoal gray, teal, turquoise.

Light
Colors that are medium to light and are neither too warm nor too cool. Sky blue, rose, pink, coral, blue-gray.

Bright
Clear, primary colors that are neither too warm nor too cool. True red, true blue, true green, hot turquoise, coral-pink.

Muted
Soft, blended colors that are neither too warm nor too cool. Mauve, jade green, grayed green, cocoa, rose, grayed blue.

Warm
Colors that reflect a golden tone. Pumpkin, gold, moss green, rust, brown.

Cool
Colors that reflect an ash, gray, or blue tone. Blue-red, slate, fuchsia, hot pink, royal blue, burgundy.

See the color charts on pages 57 - 62.

YOUR PERSONAL COLORING CHARACTERISTICS

Just as individual colors can be identified by their dominant color characteristic, so can your coloring. And just as all colors cannot be clearly divided into warm or cool, so it is with people. Therefore, let's look at some descriptions of personal coloring characteristics and see how you can describe your coloring in general color terms.

DEEP

The "deep" characteristic is the easiest to see. Do you have dark hair and eyes? If so, you're deep. How deep? Your hair color will range from black to deep brown, from a chestnut or auburn color to blue- black. Your eyes are also deep — dark brown, brown-black, deep hazel or dark olive.

Although your skintone is generally a beige, it may be olive or bronze. There are either warm or cool undertones in your skintone or a neutral tone with a mixture of warm and cool. If you are deep you can successfully wear deep colors that are not too blue or gold.

LIGHT

If your coloring can be described as "light," your hair is blond — golden or ash — medium to light. Your hair may darken when not exposed to sunlight and then rapidly lighten when bleached by the sun. Your skintone is medium to light and may appear peach or rosy. There is little contrast between your hair color and your skintone. Your eye color is gray, green, or a combination. Your eyes are not brown, deep hazel or deep blue. If you are light you can successfully wear colors that are medium to light in depth, neither too warm or too cool, nor too bright or too muted.

BRIGHT

The "bright" person has a crisp, clear look derived from a strong contrast between skin and hair color and the jewel-like clarity of the eye color. Two types of coloring can be called "bright."

The first is the person whose hair color contrasts sharply with her skintone. Your hair color is dark brown, sometimes even black or ash brown. Your skin color is almost transparent — ivory or porcelain. Accompanying this contrast in skin and hair color: bright, clear eye color in jewel tones — blue, green, turquoise or violet. They are not dark brown. This type of bright person has often been confused with the "deep." The brightness of the eyes alone demands a balance of clarity that is lost with colors that are too deep.

The second type of bright coloring, which has less contrast in hair and skintone, includes those whose eye color is true and jewel-like, blue, green, turquoise, etc. Your skintone is a bit more golden and your hair not as deep; eyebrows and lashes will be dark. If your coloring can be described as bright you can successfully wear colors that are clear — primary colors — that are neither too deep nor too light.

MUTED

When we refer to "muted" persons, we are talking about those whose coloring seems to have been toned down or softened. Interestingly, grayed-down or muted colors have a weightiness or richness about them that produces a less delicate look than light colors do, but without being dark.

Muted coloring has strength, but not depth. Your hair color is light, ash blond, or medium ash brown or blond. Your skintone ranges from golden to beige to ivory, often with an absence of any cheek color. Your eyes will be brown, hazel, teal or gray-blue. The main difference between those of you who are muted and those who are light is your eye color, which adds richness to your overall coloring—hazel, teal, turquoise, instead of light blue or green, etc. The color range is not light or dark, but medium in depth. There will, in fact, be a balance which results in a kind of "no color" look. If your coloring can be described as muted you will successfully wear softened colors of medium intensity.

WARM

The "warm" person projects a total golden glow. You have true, golden undertones in your hair, eyes and skintone. Your hair is red, auburn, golden blond, yellow-brown or strawberry. You may, in fact, have been called a redhead at some point. Your eye color is hazel, green, teal, brown, or topaz. A ruddy earthtone with gold or green combinations is projected in your eye color. Your skintone is bronze, golden beige, ivory and you often have freckles. In general, your warm coloring is medium in depth, neither very light nor very dark.

If you can describe your coloring as "warm" you will always be successful wearing warm-based colors of medium depth. See your Safe Color chart.

COOL

A "cool" person often has a rose or pink complexion. It is often described as soft or dusty. (Don't confuse this with peach coloring or a high red color). Cool coloring, in general, is in the mid-tone range, not really dark or light.

Your hair color is ash brown, dark brown, or deep ash blond. Your hair may have some warm highlights, but they are not obvious or easily seen. Overall, an ash color is projected. Remember, everyone's hair has some red highlights. In the cool person these are subtle. As our hair grays it loses pigment and becomes more ash-colored. Our appearance often softens.

Your skintone is beige, rose-beige, pink or taupe, and often projects a blue or gray undertone. Your eye color will be blue-gray, gray-blue, or cool green. If brown, it is rosy or gray-brown.

If your coloring is best described as cool, you can successfully wear cool-based colors that are neither too dark nor light. See your Safe Color chart.

Charts are included for African-American and Asian coloring as well as coloring appropriate to each type of coloring.

Which color characteristics describe you best?

To determine your dominant color characteristic, use the following charts. Identify the group that best describes your hair, eye color and skintone. *You may find that your coloring falls into two categories.* These will be closely related and have some common colors.

Examples:	**Deep**	**Bright**
	Dark hair	Dark hair
	Hazel eyes	Light hazel eyes
	Beige skin	Light skin

True red, blue, green and turquoise are some of the common colors in both the deep and bright categories. You will notice that overall the bright colors are a little more delicate than the deep. The deep contain a few stronger rich tones like teal, mahogany and brown. Let your preference and the strength of your coloring and your personality guide you.

Look at the models and the color palettes for each. Which ones do you like? Which ones bring you the most complements when you wear them?

First, select the category that best describes your coloring, but then allow your preferences to guide you in selecting a secondary, similar palette that you can work with by varying your makeup, accessories or degree of flamboyance.

If your personality is more dramatic — and the light palette best describes your physical characteristics — choose the bright as your primary color palette, reserving the light colors for times when you want a softer look.

Colors with the same or similar dominant color characteristics will always be complementary. And when you combine colors to create this overall characteristic you will be assured of a foundation of colors for your personal palette.

WEARING ALL COLORS

And remember, you can wear any and every color as long as you:

1. Combine it with one of your basic or most complementary colors.

2. Are able to use the correct makeup color range.

3. Have the desire and personality to wear the color with confidence.

Note: It is important to remember that each of us can expand our palette by adding colors according to our preferences and the latest fashion colors.

New fashion colors are provided in the *Always In Style Portfolio* each season. Ordering information appears in the back of the book.

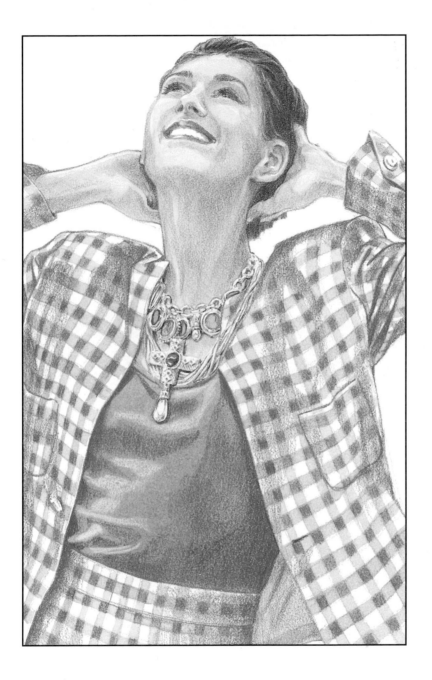

If you were to choose a checked suit which color would you select?

A **Deep** color?
A **Light** color?
A **Muted** color?
A **Bright** color?
A **Warm** color?
A **Cool** color?

DEEP

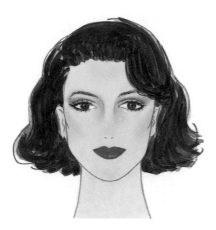

The Deep colors are medium to deep in range and are neither too warm nor too cool. Notice the strength and richness of the color.

Debra has dark brown hair and eyes, and beige skin. The Deep colors complement the strength projected by her coloring and provide the contrast necessary to accent her skintone, hair, and eyes.

Debra may add warmer or cooler colors depending on her preference, as long as she creates contrast by using her basic deep colors.

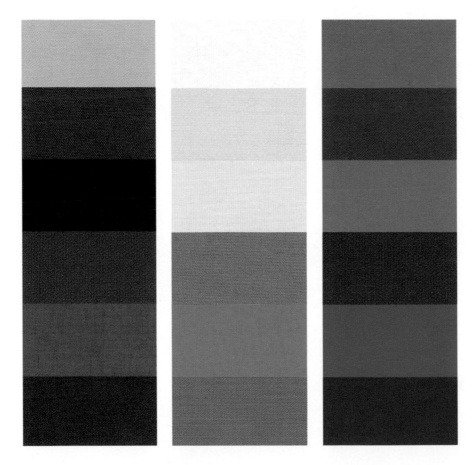

Taupe	White	Emerald Green
Charcoal Gray	Icy Blue	Forest Green
Black	Lemon Yellow	Clear Bright Warm Pink
Mahogany	Periwinkle	Wine
True Blue	Chinese Blue	True Red
Navy	Teal	Purple

LIGHT

The Light colors are light to medium in range and are neither too warm nor too cool. Notice the tone and clarity projected.

Sharon has blond hair, light blue-green eyes and beige skin. The Light colors complement her coloring and provide just enough contrast to enhance her hair, skintone, and eyes.

Sharon may add some warmer or cooler colors to her basic palette depending on her preference and the fashion trends.

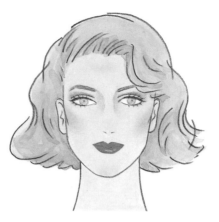

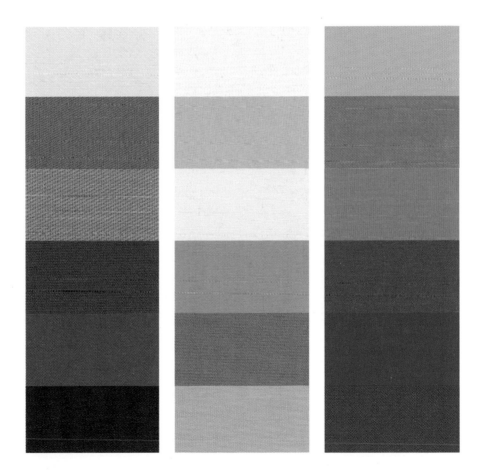

Rose Beige	**Soft White**	**Medium Blue-green**
Cocoa	**Powder Pink**	**Emerald Turquoise**
Blue-gray	**Buff**	**Clear Bright Warm Pink**
Charcoal Blue-gray	**Sky Blue**	**Rose**
True Blue	**Periwinkle**	**Watermelon**
Navy	**Turquoise**	**Medium Violet**

BRIGHT

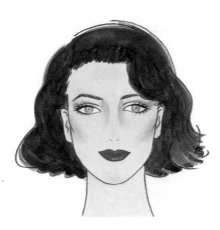

The Bright colors are medium to deep in range and are neither too warm nor too cool. Notice the jewel-like quality of the colors.

Pegeen has dark brown hair, light skin and bright green eyes. The Bright colors provide the clear contrast necessary to enhance her skintone, eyes, and haircolor.

Pegeen may add some warmer or cooler colors as long as she maintains contrast and clarity.

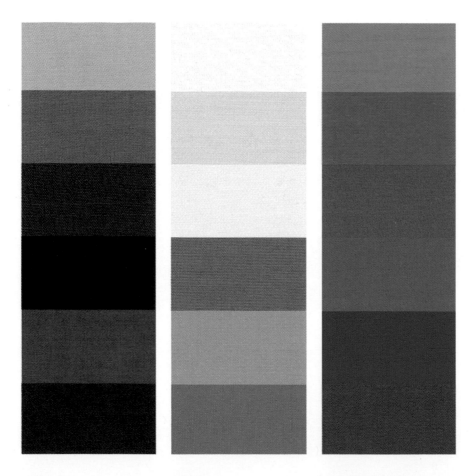

Taupe	White	Emerald Turquoise
True Gray	Icy Blue	Emerald Green
Charcoal Gray	Lemon Yellow	Magenta
Black	Periwinkle Blue	Clear Bright Warm Pink
True Blue	Bright Turquoise	True Red
Navy	Chinese Blue	Medium Violet

MUTED

The Muted colors are dusty and blended. They appear neither too warm nor too cool and are medium in depth. Notice the soft richness projected.

Karolyn has soft hazel eyes, ash-brown hair and a beige skintone. The Muted colors create a perfect balance to enhance the neutral tones of her coloring.

Karolyn may add some warm or cool colors as long as they are soft and blended.

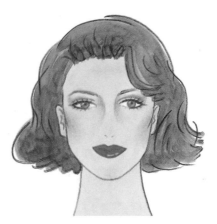

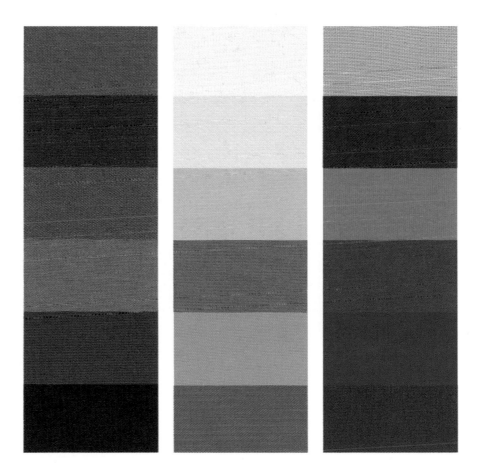

Rose Brown	Soft White	Grayed Green
Chocolate Brown	Rose Beige	Forest Green
Olive	Gold	Coral
Blue-gray	Periwinkle	Rose
Charcoal Blue-gray	Turquoise	Watermelon
Navy	Teal	Purple

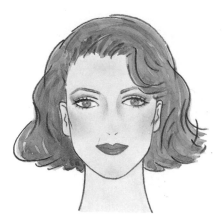

WARM

The Warm colors are medium in range and project a golden quality. Notice the richness projected by the warm undertone.

Pete has auburn hair, warm hazel eyes and golden skin. The Warm colors accent the red in her hair and the rich green in her eyes.

Pete may add some deeper or lighter colors, depending on her preferences, as long as she combines them with some golden accents.

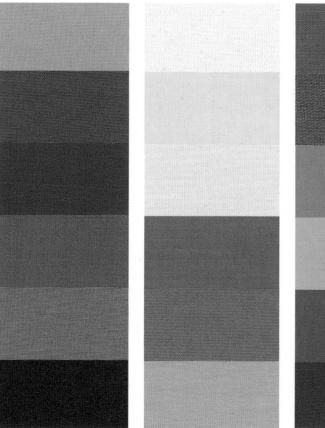

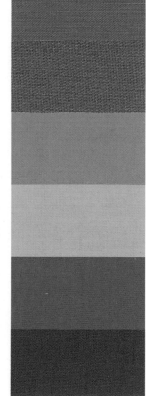

Camel	Ivory	Teal
Golden Brown	Peach	Deep Yellow-green
Rust	Yellow Gold	Coral
Moss	Terra Cotta	Salmon
Warm Gray	Periwinkle	Orange-red
Navy	Turquoise	Purple

COOL

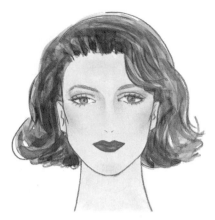

The Cool colors are medium in range and project a cool quality. Notice the subtle softness projected by the blue undertones.

Jackie has a rosy complexion, ash hair and gray-blue eyes. The Cool colors provide just enough contrast to create a balance and harmony with her hair, eyes, and skintone.

Jackie may add some deeper or lighter colors, depending on her preferences, as long as she maintains an overall cool quality.

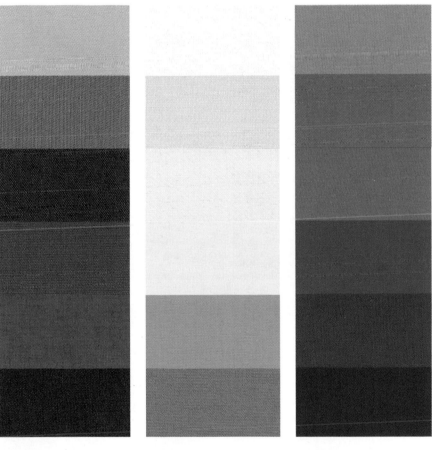

Taupe	White	Emerald Turquoise
Cocoa	Icy Blue	Emerald Green
Charcoal Gray	Icy Pink	Magenta
Charcoal Blue-gray	Light Lemon Yellow	Raspberry
Royal blue	Sky Blue	Burgundy
Navy	Periwinkle Blue	Purple

FASHION COLORS

Each season new colors appear on the fashion scene. There are always neutrals, brights, pastels, and deep rich tones. A few colors and combinations dominate and make silhouettes look fresh and new.

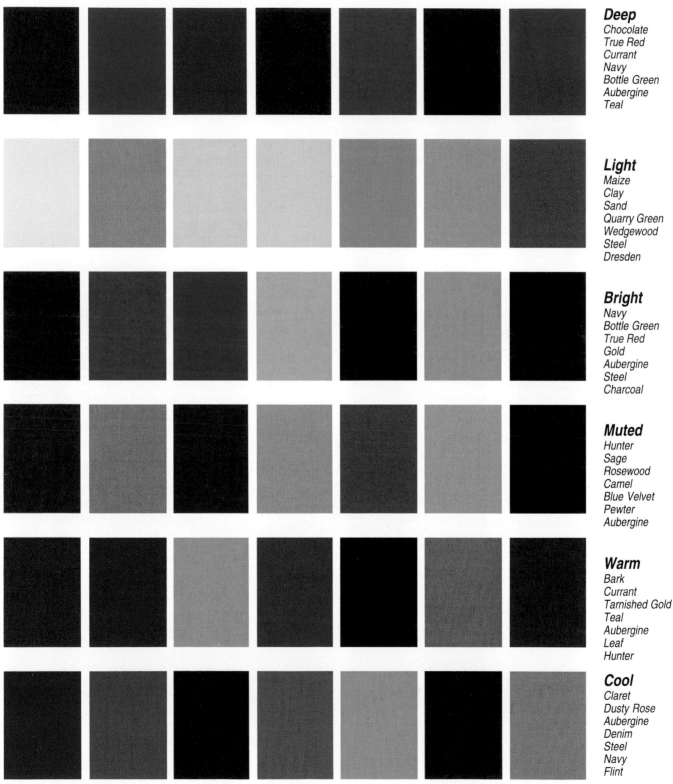

Deep
Chocolate
True Red
Currant
Navy
Bottle Green
Aubergine
Teal

Light
Maize
Clay
Sand
Quarry Green
Wedgewood
Steel
Dresden

Bright
Navy
Bottle Green
True Red
Gold
Aubergine
Steel
Charcoal

Muted
Hunter
Sage
Rosewood
Camel
Blue Velvet
Pewter
Aubergine

Warm
Bark
Currant
Tarnished Gold
Teal
Aubergine
Leaf
Hunter

Cool
Claret
Dusty Rose
Aubergine
Denim
Steel
Navy
Flint

CAUCASIAN COLORING CHARACTERISTICS

DEEP
Strong Contrast (Vivid Coloring)

Hair: Dark: black to deep brown, chestnut, auburn; may have some warm undertones.

Eyes: Deep: brown, brown-black, hazel, rich green or olive, not blue.

Skin: Beige, olive, bronze.

Recommended Colors

Soft white
Navy
Deep brown
Turquoise
Blue
Purple

Black
Charcoal gray
Taupe
True blue-teal
Mahogany

* Wear any color if combined with a deep recommended color.

LIGHT
Soft Delicate Fair Coloring

Hair: Most often blond: light to dark, ash or golden.

Eyes: Blue, blue-green, green, aqua: not deep hazel or brown.

Skin: Light: ivory to soft beige, pink, or peach; little contrast.

Recommended Colors

Soft white
Grayed navy
Blue-green
Turquoise
Periwinkle
Charcoal blue gray

Cocoa
Warm gray
Light to medium blue
Coral pinks
Watermelon
Light to medium pink-oranges

* Wear any color if combined with a recommended light to medium color.

CAUCASIAN COLORING CHARACTERISTICS

BRIGHT
Contrast in Color of Hair and Skintone

Hair: Medium to dark: brown, from ash to golden, black.

Eyes: Bright and clear: blue, blue-green, turquoise, steel gray, light hazel.

Skin: Light: ivory, porcelain or beige; translucent quality.

Recommended Colors

Soft white	Taupe
Gray	Navy
Medium blue	Periwinkle
Aqua	Turquoise
True red	True blue
True green	Bright coral
Bright pink	Violet

Wear any color if combined with a bright recommended color.

Recommended colors are from the Winter (cool) and Spring (warm) palettes.

MUTED
Medium Intensity in Coloring; Neutral Look - Medium Depth

Hair: Medium range: medium ash brown to dark ash blond.

Eyes: Grayed green, hazel, brown-green, brown, (medium to dark) green or teal.

Skin: Ivory, beige, bronze, golden — freckles and ruddiness common.

Recommended Colors

Soft white	Teal
Taupe	Turquoise
Cocoa	Rust
Rose brown	Mahogany
Blue-green	Watermelon
Grayed green	Medium green
Salmon	Warm pink
Periwinkle	

Wear any color if combined with a muted recommended color.

Recommended colors are from the Summer (cool) and Autumn (warm) palettes.

CAUCASIAN COLORING CHARACTERISTICS

WARM
Total Golden Glow (Medium Intensity)

Hair: Medium range: blond or brown with gold, red or strawberry highlights.

Eyes: Warm: green, hazel, brown, topaz, blue-green, teal.

Skin: Golden: beige, ivory, bronze; may have freckles

Recommended Colors

Ivory	Rust
Beige	Mahogany
Camel	Coral
Warm gray	Yellow
Marine navy	Golden brown
Peach	Teal-turquoise
Periwinkle	Warm red
Warm green	

* Wear any color if combined with a golden tone.

Recommended colors are from the Autumn (deep) and Spring (light) palettes.

COOL
Medium Intensity in Color (Softer Look)

Hair: Ash brown, (dark to medium) silver or salt and pepper.

Eyes: Cool: rose-brown, gray-brown, gray-blue.

Skin: Cool: beige, rose-beige, pink.

Recommended Colors

Soft white	Lavender
Gray	Burgundy
Navy	Taupe
Cocoa	Blue-red
Blue-green	Blue
Pink	Plum

* Wear any color if combined with a medium cool tone.

Recommended colors are from the Winter (deep) and Summer (light) palettes.

AFRICAN-AMERICAN COLORING CHARACTERISTICS

DEEP
Strong Contrast (Vivid Coloring)

Hair: Black, brown-black.

Eyes: Black, brown-black, red-brown, brown.

Skin: Blue-black, deep brown, rose-brown, mahogany, bronze.

Recommended Colors

Soft White	Black
Navy	Charcoal gray
Deep brown	Taupe
Turquoise	True blue-teal
Blue	Mahogany
Purple	

* Wear any color if combined with a deep recommended color.

LIGHT
Soft Delicate Fair Coloring

Hair: Soft black, brown-black, light brown, red-brown, ash brown.

Eyes: Soft black, brown, rose-brown.

Skin: Light brown, caramel, rose-beige, cocoa.

Recommended Colors

Soft white	Cocoa
Grayed navy	Warm gray
Blue-green	Light to medium blue
Turquoise	Coral pink
Periwinkle	Watermelon
Charcoal blue gray	Light to medium pink-oranges

* Wear any color if combined with a recommended light to medium color.

AFRICAN-AMERICAN COLORING CHARACTERISTICS

BRIGHT
Contrast in Color of Hair and Skintone

Hair: Black, brown-black, ash brown.

Eyes: Black, brown-black.

Skin: Light-medium brown, deep beige, cocoa, caramel.

Recommended Colors

Soft white	Taupe
Gray	Navy
Medium blue	Periwinkle
Aqua	Turquoise
True red	True blue
True green	Bright coral
Bright pink	Violet

* Wear any color if combined with a bright recommended color.

MUTED
Medium Intensity in Coloring; Neutral Look - Medium Depth

Hair: Brown, ash brown, brown-black.

Eyes: Brown-black, black, gray-brown, hazel, rose-brown.

Skin: Light brown, cocoa, rose-brown, beige; opaque, freckles, absence of strong color.

Recommended Colors

Soft white	Teal
Taupe	Turquoise
Cocoa	Rust
Rose brown	Mahogany
Blue-green	Watermelon
Grayed green	Medium green
Salmon	Warm pink
Periwinkle	

* Wear any color if combined with a muted recommended color.

AFRICAN-AMERICAN COLORING CHARACTERISTICS

WARM
Total Golden Glow (Medium Intensity)

Hair: Brown, golden brown, brown-black, chestnut.

Eyes: Warm brown, topaz, deep brown, hazel.

Skin: Bronze, caramel, mahogany, golden brown, light brown, brown; freckles.

Recommended Colors

Ivory	Rust
Beige	Mahogany
Camel	Coral
Warm gray	Yellow
Marine navy	Golden brown
Peach	Teal-turquoise
Periwinkle	Warm red
Warm green	

* Wear any color if combined with a golden tone.

COOL
Medium Intensity In Coloring (Softer Look)

Hair: Black, ash brown, blue-black.

Eyes: Brown-black, black, gray-brown, rose-brown.

Skin: Rose-brown, gray-brown, cocoa, dark brown, soft blue-black.

Recommended Colors

Soft white	Lavender
Gray	Burgundy
Navy	Taupe
Cocoa	Blue-red
Blue-green	Blue
Pink	Plum

* Wear any color if combined with a medium cool tone.

ASIAN COLORING CHARACTERISTICS

DEEP
Strong Contrast (Vivid Coloring)

Hair: Blue-black, black, brown-black, chestnut, dark brown.

Eyes: Black, brown-black, red-brown.

Skin: Olive, bronze, beige.

Recommended Colors

Soft white	Black
Navy	Charcoal gray
Deep brown	Taupe
Turquoise	True blue-teal
Blue	Mahogany
Purple	

* Wear any color if combined with a deep recommended color.

LIGHT
Soft Delicate Fair Coloring

Hair: Brown-black, ash brown, brown, soft black.

Eyes: Red-brown, brown-black, black, gray-black, golden brown.

Skin: Rose-beige, ivory, pink, peach, beige.

Recommended Colors

Soft white	Cocoa
Grayed navy	Warm gray
Blue-green	Light to medium blue
Turquoise	Coral pink
Periwinkle	Watermelon
Charcoal blue gray	Light to medium pink-oranges

* Wear any color if combined with a recommended light to medium color.

ASIAN COLORING CHARACTERISTICS

BRIGHT
Contrast in Color of Hair and Skintone

Hair: Black, brown-black, dark brown.

Eyes: Black, brown-black, hazel.

Skin: Ivory, porcelain.

Recommended Colors

Soft white	Taupe
Gray	Navy
Medium blue	Periwinkle
Aqua	True blue
True red	Bright coral
True green	Violet
Bright Pink	

* Wear any color if combined with a bright recommended color.

MUTED
Medium Intensity In Coloring; Neutral Look - Medium Depth

Hair: Brown, mahogany, ash brown, soft black.

Eyes: Brown, rose-brown, hazel, brown-black, gray-brown.

Skin: Beige, rose-beige, bronze; absence of color; opaque, freckles.

Recommended Colors

Soft white	Teal
Taupe	Turquoise
Cocoa	Rust
Rose brown	Mahogany
Blue-green	Watermelon
Grayed green	Medium green
Salmon	Warm pink
Periwinkle	

* Wear any color if combined with a muted recommended color.

ASIAN COLORING CHARACTERISTICS

WARM
Total Golden Glow (Medium Intensity)

Hair: Golden brown, auburn, dark brown, chestnut.

Eyes: Warm brown, brown-black, hazel, deep brown, topaz.

Skin: Golden beige, ivory, bronze; freckles.

Recommended Colors

Ivory	Rust
Beige	Mahogany
Camel	Coral
Warm gray	Yellow
Marine navy	Golden brown
Peach	Teal-turquoise
Periwinkle	Warm red
Warm green	

* Wear any color if combined with a golden tone.

COOL
Medium Intensity In Coloring (Softer Look)

Hair: Black, blue-black, brown-black, ash brown, dark brown, salt and pepper.

Eyes: Black, gray-brown, rose-brown.

Skin: Pink, rose-beige, gray-beige; sometimes sallow.

Recommended Colors

Soft white	Lavender
Gray	Burgundy
Navy	Taupe
Cocoa	Blue-red
Blue-green	Blue
Pink	Plum

* Wear any color if combined with a medium cool tone.

Are you
more classic,
more natural, or
more dramatic
or does it
depend on
your mood?

The
Well-Dressed Woman
wears clothes
that reflect
who she is.

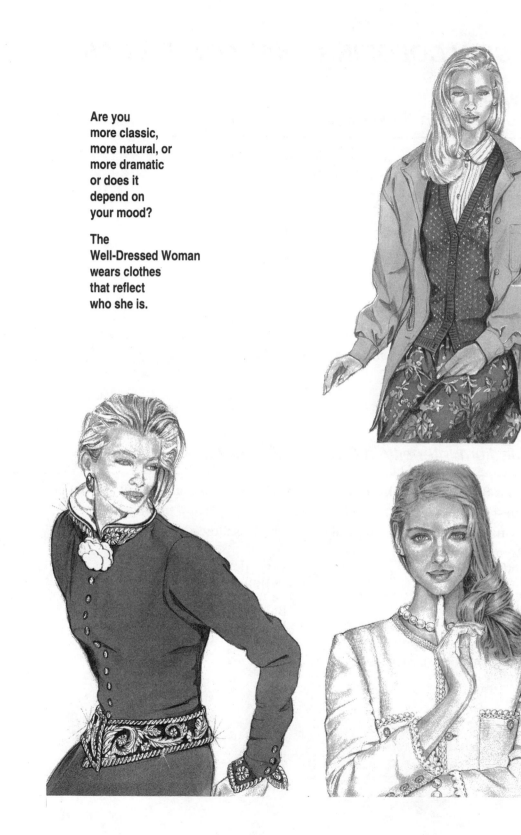

CHAPTER FIVE

Personality

The Well-Dressed Woman Wears Clothes That Express Her Personality

We have seen what a difference it makes when you wear clothes, colors and shapes that complement you physically. However, you must also be comfortable. And your clothes must reflect who you are as a unique individual inside as well as outside.

Should all those with curved bodies where the same outfit? Let's consider Madonna and Jane Pauley with respect to shape. They both have curved bodies. They do not have the same personalities.

Technically, they should be able to wear the same things. They would fit correctly *and* with freshly scrubbed skin, no makeup and hair pulled back, a softly shaped wrap dress would be fine.

Yet, Madonna in such a conservative outfit would overpower her clothes. Her personality dominates. She must exaggerate her colors and/or her shapes and proportions so that her clothes look like they are really hers.

Jane Pauley in a 16" mini skirt, exposed midriff and curved plunging top, even at a cocktail party, would look and probably feel outrageous.

At different stages of our lives we may be more or less conservative, or a little more or less daring. Because of these transitions, we should be able to adjust the way we wear our clothes to reflect who we are at any given time. There are also times when we may need to look more or less powerful than we are and that is okay, too.

How can we express our personality in the way we dress?

Very simply — through the use of accessories, details, proportions and colors we create a more exaggerated fashion forward look or a more conservative one.

For a more dramatic look:

Increase the size and scale of your accessories. Add larger earrings, a big scarf, a new shape handbag or a big pin. Use several strands of pearls or chains, or combine the two.

Shorten or lengthen a skirt a little more for an exaggerated look.

Try a more exaggerated hairstyle — asymmetrical or a new shape.

Select lipstick or eyeshadow in one of the season's new fashion colors. Emphasize either your eyes or your lips.

Mix color combinations in exciting and unique ways, using two or more color group.

For a more conservative look:

Select accessories that are restrained both in size and scale.

Shorten or lengthen a skirt just a little for a more fashionable look. Avoid extremes but be sure that your length is not outdated.

Update your hairstyle just a little. Add a wispy bang, some highlights or try a new shape.

Try a new lipstick or eyeshadow, adding just a little more emphasis to either your lips or eyes to create a more current look.

Use more neutral colors, accenting with one color.

NOTE: Keep in mind that there are not just two looks — conservative or high fashion. There are many steps along the way. Try a little larger earring, a new hairstyle and some eyeliner. If you like it, try a little more. Keep reaching in a fashion direction according to your comfort level. Over time you may find yourself moving to a more conservative or more high fashion direction according to your lifestyle and experiences. But whatever direction you choose, take care to avoid two extremes — the outdated look or that of a fashion victim.

DETERMINING YOUR CLOTHING PERSONALITY

It is important to determine whether you are more dramatic, more conservative or somewhere in between. To discover your Fashion Personality ask yourself these following questions:

UPDATE QUESTIONS

Answer **Yes** or **No**

1. Are you outgoing and extroverted?
2. Do you like to try a new hairstyles?
3. Do you love the unexpected?
4. Do you enjoy being noticed?
5. Do you think of yourself as sophisticated?
6. Do you really love clothes?
7. Are you conservative and cautious?
8. Have you worn the same or a similar hairstyle for several years?
9. Are you satisfied with your current wardrobe?
10. Do you wear only a little makeup?
11. Do you keep your skirt length about the same year after year?
12. Are you shy or reserved?

If you answered yes to the first six questions, you're ready for a high fashion or more dramatic look. If you answered yes to the last six you are more conservative but still want to strive for a fashionable look.

If your answers were mixed you probably won't want to start with an exaggerated look but are interested in reaching in a high fashion direction. Consult the *Always In Style Portfolio* for a variety of styles that can be blended to create your best look.

The well-dressed woman always wears clothes that are appropriate for the occasion.

Your wardrobe
should take you
from work
to play
to evening
with just a few
key pieces
that
mix and match
perfectly.

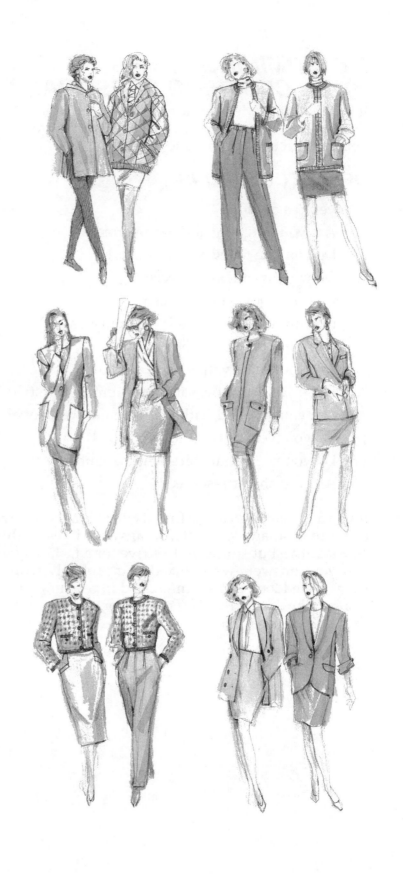

CHAPTER SIX

Your Wardrobe

A Wardrobe Appropriate For Every Occasion

Although you may have a preference for one style — romantic, natural, classic, etc., it is important that you understand the need for clothes for all occasions. We all need casual clothes, conservative business clothes (if appropriate for our job or lifestyle), and clothes for special occasions. A complementary and flexible wardrobe will enable you to have a romantic, casual and professional look.

Planning your wardrobe effectively:

1. Determine what types of clothes you need for your lifestyle. Divide your own pie into segments that reflect your lifestyle.

2. Make a list of the clothes, shoes and accessories you bought last season and roughly add up the cost of each item. Add between 10 and 15 percent to get this season's clothing costs. Use this to determine the season's budget based upon your personal goals.

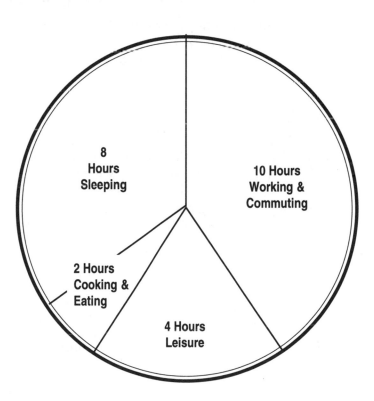

8 Hours Sleeping

10 Hours Working & Commuting

2 Hours Cooking & Eating

4 Hours Leisure

3. Experiment with the cost-per-wearing formula below. Remember that for wise investment-buying you can spend more on the items that you will be wearing more often. Let's say you buy a two-piece dress for $100.00 that you will wear every two weeks for 26 wearings. Divide $100.00 by 26 and your formula will look like this:

$$\frac{\$100.00}{26} = \$3.85 \text{ per wearing}$$

Compare this with a cocktail dress costing $150.00 and worn 5 times. The formula will look like this:

$$\frac{\$150.00}{5} = \$30.00 \text{ per wearing}$$

4. Review the wardrobe chart appropriate for your body line in this chapter to help you create a capsule wardrobe. You may find purchasing a capsule wardrobe both time-saving and more economical in the long run.

CAPSULE WARDROBE

Now that you know the shapes and colors that complement you and how to accessorize your outfits to express your personality, you can create a wardrobe that will take you from play to work to evening with a very few pieces.

Use the following suggestions to help you plan your capsule wardrobe. A few pieces in your correct shape and color will work together to create many complementary outfits. Select 10 to 14 pieces; these will create up to 30 different outfits.

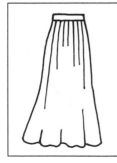

Jacket (can be suit jacket)
* Solid neutral color
* Classic style in your line
* Matching buttons or no buttons
* Natural or quality blend fabric
* Quality tailoring

2nd Jacket (Optional)
(complementary color; or pattern to work with 1st jacket)

Essential Accessories
* For day in neutral color pumps or slingbacks
* Flat or sport shoe
* Bag
* Good walking shoes or sports shoe
* Boots for winter (optional)
* 3 scarves
* Earrings
* Bracelet
* Necklace

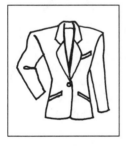

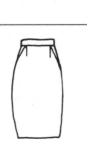

2 Skirts
* Match jacket above or
* Match 2nd jacket or contrast with neutral, solid, tweed, herringbone or check

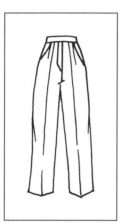

Pants
* Solid neutral
* Quality fabric and tailoring

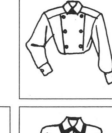

First Blouse
* White, soft white, ivory or oyster
* Simple style

Second Blouse
* Any solid color
* Print or pattern
* Front button for use as overblouse

Third Blouse
* Solid color
* More dressy style and fabric

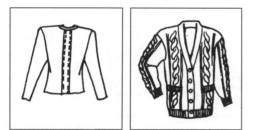

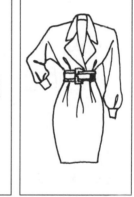

Two Sweaters and/or Knit Tops
* Basic color
* Cardigan style will work as jacket
* Crew, cowl, V, turtleneck
* Cotton knit in summer

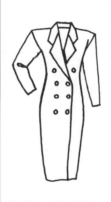

Dress I
* Solid color
* Simple style for day or night
* Minimum detail
* Long sleeve

Dress II
(optional)
* Two-piece
* Print or pattern

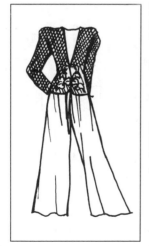

Evening Pants, Skirt or Dress
* Basic color for pants or skirt
* Any color in your palette
* Dressy fabric

Evening Dress
(if necessary)
* Any color
* Two-piece for versatility

Casual Wear
* leggings, jeans, big shirt, sweater, turtleneck, jacket/parka
* Fun colors or prints
* Casual fabric

Coat - all weather, winter
* Neutral color
* Quality fabric and tailoring
* Simple, classic style
* Matching buttons
* May be all-weather fabric

CAPSULE: STRAIGHT

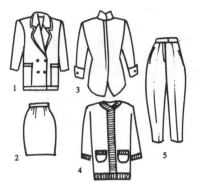

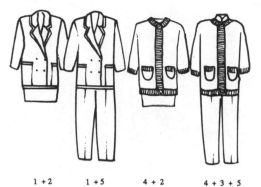

1. Solid Neutral Jacket
2. Simple Matching Skirt
3. Solid Classic Blouse
4. Cardigan Style Sweater
5. Neutral Classic Trouser

1 + 2   1 + 5   4 + 2   4 + 3 + 5

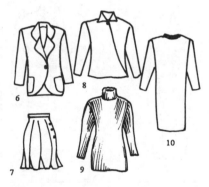

6. Second Jacket (may be check, plaid, tweed or contrasting neutral
7. Contrasting or Matching Skirt
8. Colored Blouse (may be print or dressy fabric
9. Knit Top
10. Simple Classic Dress for day or evening

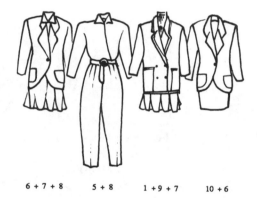

6 + 7 + 8   5 + 8   1 + 9 + 7   10 + 6

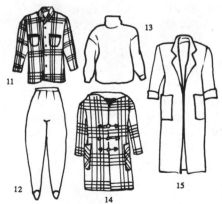

11. Big Shirt
12. Leggings, Stirrups or Jeans
13. Casual Crew, Cowl or Turtleneck Sweater
14. Casual Jacket or Parka
15. Simple Classic Style Coat

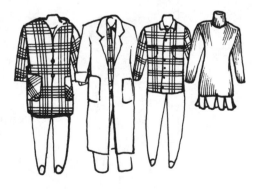

14 + 12 + 13   11 + 5 + 15   13 + 11 + 12   9 + 7

CAPSULE: SOFT STRAIGHT

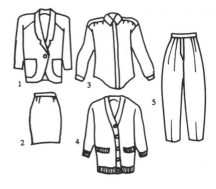

1. Solid Neutral Jacket
2. Simple Matching Skirt
3. Solid Classic Blouse
4. Knit Top
5. Neutral Classic Trouser

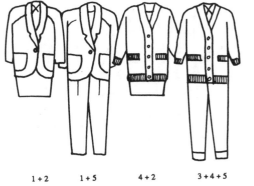

1 + 2   1 + 5   4 + 2   3 + 4 + 5

6. Second Jacket (may be check, plaid, tweed or contrasting neutral)
7. Neutral or Contrasting Skirt
8. Colored Blouse (may be print or dressy fabric)
9. Knit Top
10. Simple Classic Dress for day or evening

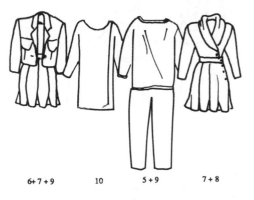

6 + 7 + 9   10   5 + 9   7 + 8

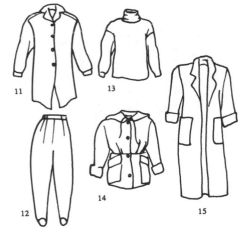

11. Big Shirt
12. Leggings, Stirrups or Jeans
13. Casual Crew, Cowl or Turtleneck
14. Casual Jacket or Parka
15. Simple Classic Style Coat

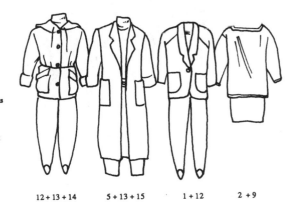

12 + 13 + 14   5 + 13 + 15   1 + 12   2 + 9

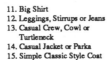

CAPSULE: STRAIGHT SOFT

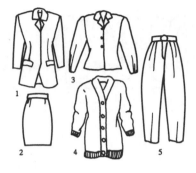

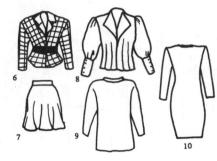

1. Solid Neutral Jacket
2. Simple Matching Skirt
3. Solid Classic Blouse
4. Cardigan Style Sweater
5. Neutral Classic Trouser

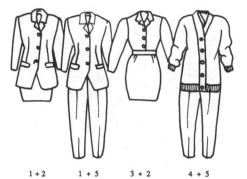

1 + 2   1 + 5   3 + 2   4 + 5

6. Second Jacket (may be check, plaid, tweed or contrasting neutral
7. Contrasting or Matching Skirt
8. Colored Blouse (may be print or dressy fabric
9. Knit Top
10. Simple Classic Dress for day or evening

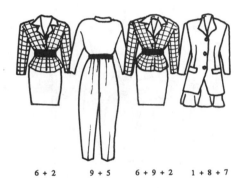

6 + 2   9 + 5   6 + 9 + 2   1 + 8 + 7

11. Big Shirt
12. Leggings, Stirrups or Jeans
13. Casual Crew, Cowl or Turtleneck
14. Casual Jacket or Parka
15. Simple Classic Style Coat

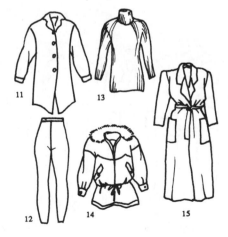

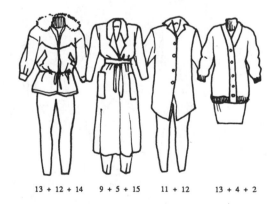

13 + 12 + 14   9 + 5 + 15   11 + 12   13 + 4 + 2

CAPSULE: CURVED

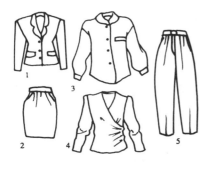

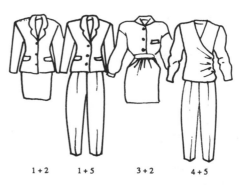

1. Solid Neutral Jacket
2. Simple Matching Skirt
3. Solid Classic Blouse
4. Knit Top
5. Neutral Classic Trouser

1 + 2   1 + 5   3 + 2   4 + 5

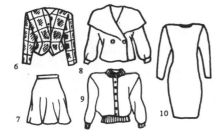

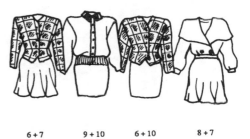

6. Second Jacket (may be check, plaid, tweed or contrasting neutral
7. Contrasting or Matching Skirt
8. Colored Blouse (may be print or dressy fabric
9. Knit Top
10. Simple Classic Dress for day or evening

6 + 7   9 + 10   6 + 10   8 + 7

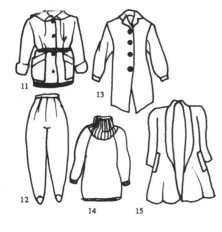

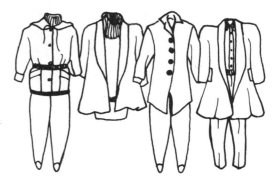

11. Big Shirt
12. Leggings, Stirrups or Jeans
13. Casual Jacket or Parka
14. Casual Crew, Cowl or Turtleneck Sweater
15. Simple Classic Style Coat

11 + 12   2 + 14 + 15   12 + 13   5 + 9 + 15

Isn't it enough
to wear clothes
that complement
you physically,
and
are appropriate
for the occasion.

If you look dated
— if you look
out of touch
with what's
going on today —
you aren't really
the
Well-Dressed
Woman.

CHAPTER SEVEN

Staying Current

The well-dressed woman is current and fashionable

Every season women are bombarded with new fashion choices. New colors, shapes, proportions and details. We recognize the need to look fashionable, but how? Where do we begin? How do we know what's new and current when everywhere we look — the store windows, magazines, displays — things are constantly changed. New merchandise appears non-stop. Just when we buy that new jacket, another one comes in. Should we have waited? What else is coming? And how should we wear the jacket? With a sweater, blouse, scarf; with a pin, pearls or chains? It all seems so difficult and confusing. Do we need to buy a new wardrobe every season?

It is really very simple when you understand fashion and fashion forecasting, and know the fashion picture. Especially when you can know all of this a whole season ahead of time.

Let's stop for a minute and look behind the scenes at fashion and fashion forecasting.

What's in fashion?

Fashion is a reflection of what's happening in society as interpreted by designers, manufacturers and buyers. The movies, theater, art exhibits, economic and political events all affect the colors and styles we see each season.

It starts with color. Each year members of the International Color Association meet to decide on the new colors that will be seen as far ahead as two years in the future. The home furnishings, automotive, appliance and fashion worlds all work together. Think about the harvest gold and avocado green appliances of the 70's, the pink and gray tile baths of the 50's.

To stay current and fashionable, we need to know the new colors and color stories and how to combine them with the basics we already have for a much newer, updated look.

After colors are selected, fabric design, silhouette shape and details are combined to reflect the designer's interpretation of what's new. Remember the bamboo motifs of the early 80's? The Mediterranean motifs of the 60's in home furnishings?

The film factor
In the fashion world, "Out of Africa" and "Crocodile Dundee" brought safari looks; "Dances With Wolves," Native American touches and "Thelma and Louise," south of the border themes. Post-war patriotism has brought touches of Americana — flag motifs and homespun fabrics. There are often several themes seen at the same time. We see a return to ultra-feminine looks reminiscent of the post war 40's combined with Americana motifs.

Designers and manufacturers often get their inspiration from movies, and from street scenes in Tokyo, Paris, Milan and St. Tropez. They know a year ahead what's going to be available in the stores and buyers buy a year or six months ahead. Retailers spend thousands of dollar a year to subscribe to services like the Tobe' Report and Nigel French that tell them the complete fashion story and recommend merchandise.

Saving time, money and indecision
It makes sense for each and every one of us to know the new colors, fabrics, themes, shapes and silhouettes a full season ahead also, so we can plan our wardrobes and our budgets.

Armed with this information, we can then update our existing wardrobes by lengthening or shortening our skirts a little; mixing the green T shirt with blue slacks this year for a new color story; tying a scarf around our waist instead of our neckline; knowing when to bring out pearls or add the great rhinestone pin you saved from 10 years ago.

You can then add a few *new* Must Haves; a lace pocket square, opaque hose, a chiffon scarf, checked jacket or new longer length jacket.

It is also important to update your hose colors and shoes. Nothing is worse than outdated suntan hose and scuffed shoes on an otherwise well-dressed woman.

And now that you know your body shape and coloring you can select the checked jacket that is the right shape for you, the new chiffon scarf in your best color, the flattering satin blouse with just the right neckline because it complements your face shape.

Predicting your fashion future

Ten years ago, I decided to put together an affordable and complete Always In Style forecast every six months — a full season ahead — to offer just this advice. June 15th is my publication date for the Fall/Winter edition and December 15th for the Spring/Summer version of this fully illustrated fashion forecast. All silhouettes are identified with body line symbols.

With your *Always In Style Portfolio* you can save both time and money each season. You learn not only the choices that will be available but which ones are right for you and new color groups in specific color categories.

Each season you will also be able to purchase some very special MUST HAVES to update your wardrobe by watching my MUST HAVES BY DORIS POOSER show on the QVC Cable Network.

Updating
your hair style
and makeup
can make
an important
difference.

Don't look
outdated
when you can
look current
and
fashionable.

CHAPTER EIGHT

The Finishing Touches

Hair and Makeup

You have learned the four steps to being a well-dressed woman of the 90's; how to select clothes that complement you physically, to wear clothes that express your personality, and to create a capsule wardrobe that provides pieces that work for all occasions, so that you can always be appropriately dressed.

And now you can be "always in style" by subscribing to the *Always In Style Portfolio* and updating your look each season.

But let's not forget to put the finishing touches on your look by updating your makeup and hairstyles as well.

From the neck down you can get a 10, but if your hair and makeup are not updated you miss the mark.

The same four steps to becoming a well-dressed woman apply to hair and makeup. The colors and shapes must complement you physically, reflect your personality and lifestyle, be appropriate for the occasion and be current and fashionable.

Makeup - Too much, too little, or poorly applied makeup all send out the wrong messages.

Too much says cheap, inexpensive, inappropriate. Think of thick pancake makeup, false eyelashes, Cleopatra eyeliner, heavy rouge and shadow. Off stage these excesses simply are less than appropriate or professional regardless of the clothes.

Too little says incomplete; lack of attention to detail, unsure, unsophisticated. There have actually been studies done by a major beauty product manufacturer that found that women in the corporate world earned 20 percent more money when they wore makeup (properly applied, of course). Obviously, there are times when little or no makeup is appropriate (exercising, sleeping, etc.).

Inappropriate or incorrectly applied color or placement says outdated, cheap, disinterested in self or unwilling to change. The frosted blue eyeshadow, Cleopatra eyes and frosted pink lipstick of the 50's do not look youthful, even though it may be the look you wore when you were young.

An amazing amount of progress has been made in the cosmetic industry in terms of quality and natural color choices in the last ten years. You can easily wear the correct color and amount of makeup for any occasion, and look natural yet "finished." And, most importantly, you will be taking care of your skin by protecting and nourishing it.

Once again, it is a matter of knowing which colors to choose and learning how to apply them.

Putting your best face forward

For your basic natural look, select makeup colors that complement your coloring. Choose lipstick and blush colors in the same range as the reds and pinks in the suggested palette or palettes for your coloring. Go deeper or brighter for evening or if you have a more sophisticated or dramatic personality — add more color, a touch of gold at the center of your lid, more liner or colored mascara for that special evening.

Each season note the new colors and techniques in the *Always In Style Portfolio* and make changes. Changes are often difficult since we are apt to become comfortable with the security of "sameness," but change is necessary and in fact is good. It generates energy, a sense of expectation, and helps you focus on the future.

Understand that your eye becomes accustomed to the frosted pink lipstick just as it does to the bell-bottom trousers, exaggerated shoulder pads, or short or long skirts after seeing these things over and over on someone else. Just as we begin to feel comfortable we start to see new colors and styles. It takes a conscious effort to make a change — even a gradual change.

So even when the frosted pink lipstick is a complementary color, when it becomes outdated it's time to try a more matte rose, or coral-pink, depending on the season. Try mixing your old shade with the newer color to gradually adjust to a new depth or look. I promise you will look younger and more alive and well-dressed.

See application charts on pages 95 - 97.

Hairstyles

Our hair is often referred to as our crowning glory and rightly so. A great hairstyle, in my opinion, should be the first step and your number-one focus. Color, shape, condition and movement all make the most difference in looking "younger."

I can often look out into the audience and tell how old a person is by the way she is wearing her hair. Remember Doris Day movies in the 50's and 60's and the bobby socks and suede loafers? It's amazing how easy it is to see how outdated somebody else can look.

Also consider the woman who is prematurely gray. Give her a wonderful cut and swingy hairstyle and her hair becomes her major asset. Gray hair in an outdated style, however says old.

With all the wonderful hair care and styling products on the market today there is little excuse for not having healthy hair that is easy to take care of in a new and fashionable style.

Complementing shapes and colors bring compliments

Select a shape that complements your face shape. Play up those angles or curves by choosing blunt, asymmetrical cuts if your face is more angular, or wispy, rounded or softer shapes for a more curved face shape.

Highlight your hair with a golden, red or honey tone to add warmth to your skintone. Add a clear, burgundy tint for a cooler tone. Remember that no one is all cool. You can create a little more warmth by adding a few highlights. Warm highlights make your hair and skintone look younger.

Natural hair color has some warm tones, especially when we're young. Look at a child in the sun. Notice hair after a perm. By adding just a few highlights you create movement, a more youthful look and can still have flexibility in your color range.

Avoid extremes in color or shape unless you have the personality and desire to express more drama or sophistication.

Update your colors and shapes. Some seasons we see more curl and others more wind-blown looks. Some years we see a more fixed look.

Save the bubble for the bath

Although some of the 60's, 70's and 40's styles are returning, we still do not want the old teased-up, bubble look of the 70's. The *Always In Style Portfolio* shows new hairstyles each season. Just a little change in color and shape really can make you look younger and certainly is the finishing touch for any well-dressed woman.

And finally, my pet peeve — overly long fingernails. While lengths vary from season to season, really long nails *never* say style and class. And fortunately, in fashion, we are seeing a movement toward shorter nails; less color for day and work is always correct. Save the colors for fun or evening.

Choose a color that complements or blends with your lipstick — it does not have to match. Keep your hands well-groomed. The importance of good grooming cannot be overstated.

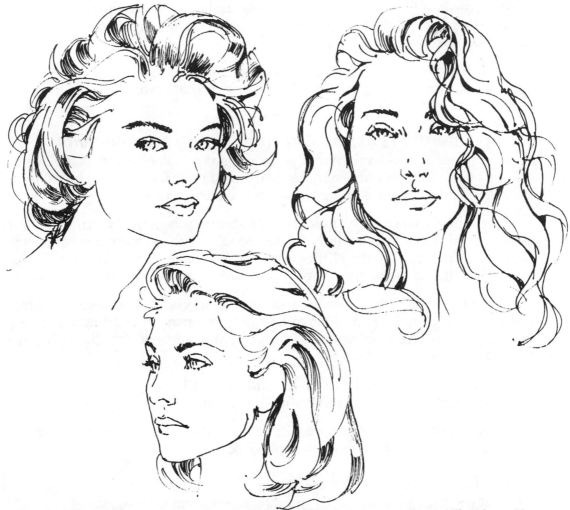

Choose a hairstyle that complements your face shape, reflects your personality and lifestyle, and is current and fashionable.

MAKEUP APPLICATION CHARTS

Just as style, colors and fashions change, so do looks in makeup. Some years eyes are emphasized, some years cheeks or lips. New colors and products are introduced each year to complement the fashion colors and themes and to help create a younger, healthier, more current look in makeup. Use the following charts as a guide only.

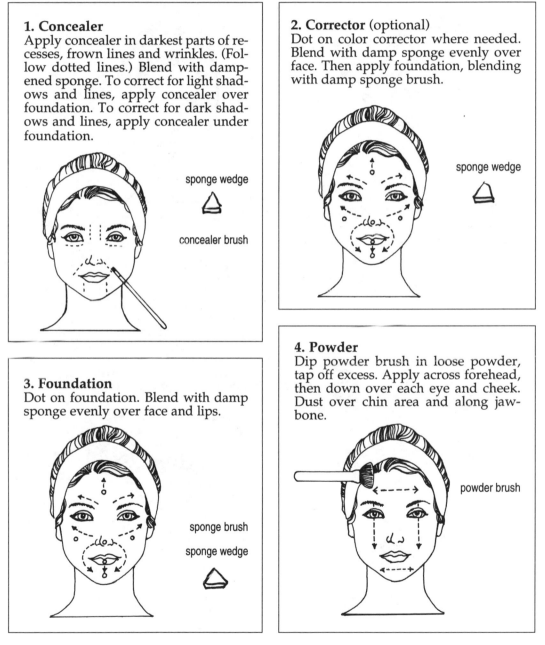

1. Concealer
Apply concealer in darkest parts of recesses, frown lines and wrinkles. (Follow dotted lines.) Blend with dampened sponge. To correct for light shadows and lines, apply concealer over foundation. To correct for dark shadows and lines, apply concealer under foundation.

sponge wedge

concealer brush

2. Corrector (optional)
Dot on color corrector where needed. Blend with damp sponge evenly over face. Then apply foundation, blending with damp sponge brush.

sponge wedge

3. Foundation
Dot on foundation. Blend with damp sponge evenly over face and lips.

sponge brush

sponge wedge

4. Powder
Dip powder brush in loose powder, tap off excess. Apply across forehead, then down over each eye and cheek. Dust over chin area and along jawbone.

powder brush

5. Blush

Apply blusher along top of cheekbone, beginning under center of eye and smooth up and out into hairline. Do not bring blusher lower than an imaginary line from bottom of nose to just under ear, or too close to eye.

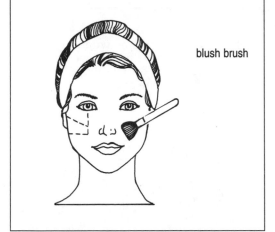

blush brush

6. Eyebrows

To shape eyebrows, line up a pencil alongside nose. This is where the eyebrow should begin. Pivot pencil over center of eye to find the peak of your arch. Then pivot pencil to outer corner of eye for the end of brow. Pluck hairs to define arch and clean brow-bone. Fill in with brow pencil where necessary.

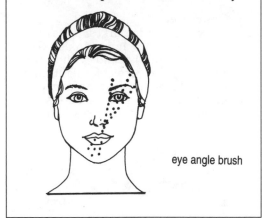

eye angle brush

7. Eyeliner

To enhance shape and size of eyes: Apply along outer edge of eye and under eye.

For little
or no lid
draw line
as shown.

For
prominent lid
draw line
as shown.

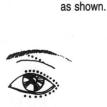

For
average lid
draw line
as shown.

8. Eyeshadow

Highlighter - Apply from lash to eyebrow to even out and lighten your lid and highlight the top of your brow bone. *Contour* - Use along the crease of your eye to lift and enhance your orbital bone. *Lid Accent* - Use accent shade on outer third of lid (see triangle) and under outer third of lower lash. Blend all together for a soft effect.

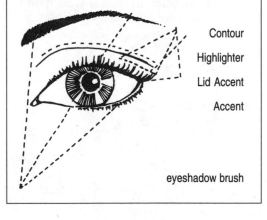

Contour

Highlighter

Lid Accent

Accent

eyeshadow brush

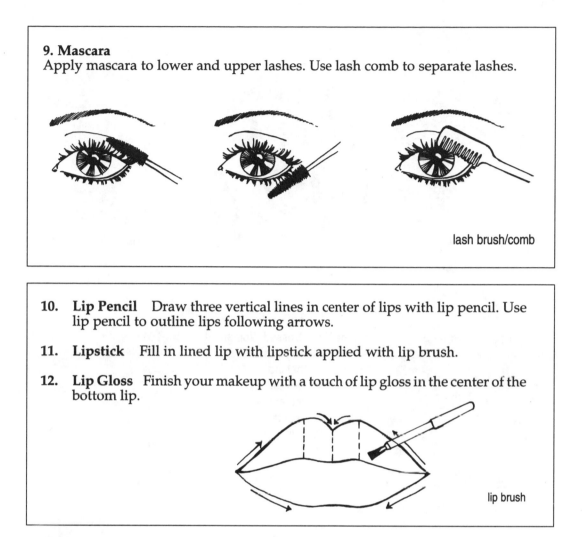

9. Mascara
Apply mascara to lower and upper lashes. Use lash comb to separate lashes.

lash brush/comb

10. **Lip Pencil**   Draw three vertical lines in center of lips with lip pencil. Use lip pencil to outline lips following arrows.

11. **Lipstick**   Fill in lined lip with lipstick applied with lip brush.

12. **Lip Gloss**   Finish your makeup with a touch of lip gloss in the center of the bottom lip.

lip brush

Evening Tips
1. Moisten a cotton ball with a mild toner. Wipe forehead, nose, and chin areas.
2. Remove any lipstick.
3. Freshen nose, forehead, chin, and lips with foundation.
4. Dust with translucent or iridescent powder.
5. Freshen eyelids with highlighter. Add a little gold shadow to the center of the lids. Touch up accent color.
6. Add a lighter shade of blush to top of cheekbones. Accent hollows of cheeks with deeper tone.
7. Reapply lipstick. Touch lip gloss or lighter shade of lipstick to center of bottom lip for a sensual look.
8. Add a second coat of "color" mascara.

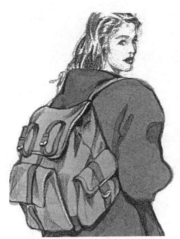
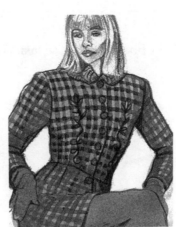
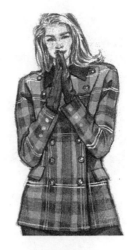

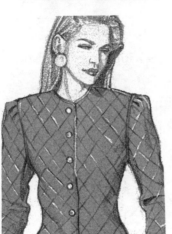

Who are you?

The Well-Dressed Woman
wears clothes
that are
an expression
of who she is,
inside
as well as out.

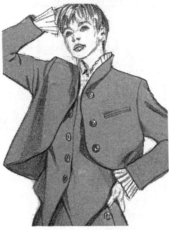

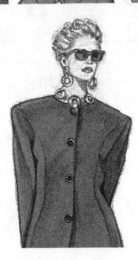
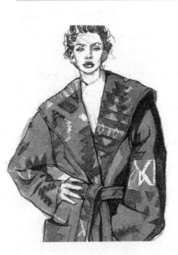
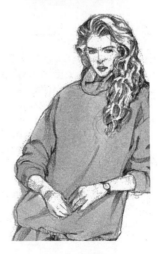

CHAPTER NINE

Your True Self

I promised you that by following the Simple Rules of Dressing that you, too, could project style and class; seem confident and assured and in control. By now you can see that it really is quite easy to become the Well-Dressed Woman of the 90's and look forward to having people say, "she's lucky, she always looks so wonderful."

But with my promise comes a word of caution and the reflection on Henry Rogers' full definition of image: "Our self-image *and* our public image."

You now know how to fix your public image. And, as Dr. Joyce Brothers says, it will certainly help your self-image. But it is not the whole story. We must also work on our self-image — our inner feelings of self — at the same time. It is okay to use our public image as a temporary crutch but beware of becoming too dependent on it. Don't allow it to become a facade — don't let it present a false front of someone other than the real you.

Making both images count

Again, I speak from experience. It was very easy for me to become comfortable with the image people saw and responded to on a business and professional level. Many doors and opportunities were opened to me because of my public image. I look credible, successful, believable and professional.

Personally and socially I found that my look of confidence, self-sufficiency and control was often interpreted to mean that I was aloof, unfriendly and unapproachable. Because at that time I really hadn't dealt directly with my "hurt" self-image, my pain, insecurities and fears, I hid behind this public image and in fact reinforced these perceptions.

The less people reached out to me, the more rejected I felt. The more aloof and distant I appeared, the lonelier and more hurt I became. My air of confidence and self-sufficiency was sending the wrong message.

I was rarely invited to parties or out to dinner. I was living in the South and people would say "stop by and see us sometime," or "we must get together." But I wouldn't just "stop over" and we never did get together. I took it personally but later heard comments like "she's too busy, always gone or can't be bothered with us."

The truth of what was happening to me started to become clear at an industry cocktail party several years ago. A colleague walked up to me and said, "You look so beautiful tonight. Your dress is lovely." Tears came to my eyes. My colleague became very uncomfortable and immediately asked me what was wrong.

I thanked her for her compliments and explained that I rarely received compliments anymore. At first she looked surprised and then said, "in all honesty, people don't compliment you because they think you know you look good and you look so confident that you don't need compliments."

Looking back to move forward

I gave a lot of thought to that comment and considered my personal life over the previous five years. I realized that, in spite of being attractive and available, I never almost got asked out for a drink, or for dinner or am even approached by men for a date. Even traveling alone to all parts of the world on airplanes, or in hotels and restaurants.

I had an opportunity the following week to ask a group of 30 professional men attending one of my seminars if they would ask me out, or start up a conversation with me. The majority said no. They said that upon first looking at me they felt intimidated and uncomfortable, and doubted that I would bother to respond.

I realized that important 55 percent of my visual first impression was presenting not my true self but only my public image. In my personal life, if I wanted to have people reach out to me, I was going to have to reach out to them and show them my true self, even though it might not be perfect. My body language and presentation and perhaps even my voice were reinforcing my image of complete control, confidence and professionalism and creating an overall impression of aloofness.

I was using my public image as a defense, hiding behind it, instead of using it as a tool because I was afraid of being rejected again, not loved, not approved of. I needed to work on accepting myself and feeling good about myself, so that people could look and say, "She is confident, self-assured and in control and I want to know her better. She is a real person with the same needs, desires and life experiences as the rest of us."

As you work on improving your personal image, remember to reach out to that Well-Dressed Woman. She's a real person, too. And as *you become the Well-Dressed Woman of the 90's, be sure to take steps to work on your self-image, and begin to present the best of your true self, your true image:*

THE IMAGE OF THE REAL WOMAN OF THE 90'S:

CONFIDENT, SELF-ASSURED AND SELF-LOVED.

MY ANSWERS TO QUESTIONNAIRE

1. List the four ways in which your clothes can complement you physically.

a) They have the same or similar shape as my body.
b) They are in a color that complements my coloring.
c) They fit properly — are elegantly loose.
d) They have been adjusted to camouflage any minor figure problems.

2. How can you express your personality in the way you dress?

a) Choose accessories in different sizes.
b) Shorten or lengthen skirts according to the fashion direction.
c) Exaggerate my hairstyle.
d) Use a more dramatic makeup application and/or color.

3. List the different occasions and types of clothes you need for your lifestyle.

Occasion	Types of Clothes
Play	Exercise clothes, swimwear, shorts, slacks, sweaters, jeans
Work	Suits, jackets, blouses, dresses
Evening *(dress)*	Cocktail dress or suit, dress pants, gown

4. List three ways to help you determine your wardrobe needs.

a) List types of activities.
b) Determine your budget.
c) Figure time spent on each activity to determine items and cost using per-wearing formula.

5. List a basic capsule wardrobe of 10 to 14 pieces that will serve all of your needs.

1 suit jacket/blazer
2 skirts
1 slack
2 knit tops or sweaters
Dress

1 coat
1 jacket
3 blouses
1 two-piece dress

6. How can you quickly change a casual outfit to make it appropriate for work or give it a dressy look?

Change accessories, shoes and bag. Change makeup.

7 . List four ways in which you can update your look each season.

a) Change hairstyle.
b) Shorten or lengthen skirt.
c) Add a new color.
d) Add a new "Must Have" from the *Always In Style Portfolio.*

8. Do you like wearing black, or want to but haven't felt confident in black? How can you wear black or any other fashion color in a way that is complementary to you?

Combine it with one of your best colors and be sure it is your right style and shape. Apply additional makeup. Add more exaggerated accessories.

9. List four makeup tips that can change your look from day to evening.

a) Add a "color" mascara to your lash tips.
b) Use a color liner on the outer edges of your eye.
c) Add gold shadow to the center of your lid.
d) Touch of lip gloss — lighter shade of lipstick on center of bottom lip for a sensual look.

10. Describe your personal style.

My personal style is a total reflection of who I am.

— *Doris Pooser*

INDEX

DORIS POOSER